A FEAST OF INFORMATION—
for people who love to eat but need to know
the carbohydrate count of their meals.

THE BARBARA KRAUS 1984
CARBOHYDRATE GUIDE TO BRAND
NAMES & BASIC FOODS lists thousands of
basic and ready-to-eat foods from appetizers
to desserts—carry it to the supermarket, to the
restaurant, to the beach, to the coffee cart,
and on trips.

Flip through these fact-filled pages. Mix, match,
and keep track of grams as they add up. But
remember, strawberry shortcake is fattening
any way you slice it!

The Barbara Kraus
1984 Carbohydrate
Guide to
Brand Names and
Basic Foods

SIGNET Books by Barbara Kraus

(0451)

☐ **CALORIES AND CARBOHYDRATES by Barbara Kraus. Revised edition.** This complete guide contains over 8,000 brand names and basic foods with their caloric and carbohydrate counts. Recommended by doctors, nutritionists, and family food planners as an indispensable aid to those who must be concerned with what they eat, it will become the most important diet reference source you will ever own.
(123301—$3.95)*

☐ **THE BARBARA KRAUS CALORIE GUIDE TO BRAND NAMES & BASIC FOODS, 1983 Edition.** Count calories with this—the most up-to-date and accurate calorie counter that lists thousands of basic and ready-to-eat foods from appetizers to desserts. (119967—$1.95)*

☐ **THE BARBARA KRAUS CARBOHYDRATE GUIDE TO BRAND NAMES & BASIC FOODS, 1983 Edition.** At a glance you'll know the carbohydrate count of many of your favorite brand name and basic foods, with this, the most up-to-date, accurate carbohydrate counter.
(119975—$1.95)*

☐ **THE BARBARA KRAUS SODIUM GUIDE TO BRAND NAME & BASIC FOODS, 1983 Edition.** This complete guide contains a feast of information for people who love to eat but need to know the sodium count of their meals. (122380—$1.95)*

☐ **THE BARBARA KRAUS DICTIONARY OF PROTEIN.** The most complete and accurate listing published of the protein and caloric count per individual serving of thousands of brand names and basic foods. (087917—$2.50)

☐ **THE BARBARA KRAUS GUIDE TO FIBER IN FOODS. Revised Edition.** Provides the best available information on the fiber and caloric content of thousands of basic and brand-name foods.
(099761—$2.50)*

*Prices slightly higher in Canada

The Barbara Kraus 1984 Carbohydrate Guide to Brand Names and Basic Foods

A SIGNET BOOK

NEW AMERICAN LIBRARY

NAL BOOKS ARE AVAILABLE AT QUANTITY DISCOUNTS
WHEN USED TO PROMOTE PRODUCTS OR SERVICES.
FOR INFORMATION PLEASE WRITE TO PREMIUM MARKETING DIVISION,
THE NEW AMERICAN LIBRARY, INC., 1633 BROADWAY,
NEW YORK, NEW YORK 10019.

Excerpted from *Dictionary of Calories and Carbohydrates*

SIGNET TRADEMARK REG. U.S. PAT. OFF. AND FOREIGN COUNTRIES
REGISTERED TRADEMARK—MARCA REGISTRADA
HECHO EN CHICAGO, U.S.A.

SIGNET, SIGNET CLASSIC, MENTOR, PLUME, MERIDIAN and NAL BOOKS
are published by The New American Library, Inc.,
1633 Broadway, New York, New York 10019

FIRST PRINTING, JANUARY, 1984

1 2 3 4 5 6 7 8 9

PRINTED IN THE UNITED STATES OF AMERICA

For Bob, Aileen,
Charles, Doreen, Robert,
and James Gildersleeve

Foreword

The composition of the foods we eat is not static: it changes from time to time. In the case of *brand-name* products, manufacturers alter their recipes to reflect the availability of ingredients, advances in technology, or improvements in formulae. Each year new products appear on the market and some old ones are discontinued.

On the other hand, information on *basic foods* such as meats, vegetables, and fruits may also change as a result of the development of better analytical methods, different growing conditions, or new marketing practices. These changes, however, are usually relatively small as compared with those in manufactured products.

Some differences may be found between the values in this book and those appearing on the product labels. This is usually due to the fact that the Food and Drug Administration permits manufacturers to round the figures reported on labels. The data in this book are reported as calculated without rounding. If large differences between the two sets of values are noted, they may be due to changes in product formulae, and in those cases the label data should be used.

For all these reasons, a book of carbohydrate or nutritive values of foods must be kept up to date by a periodic reviewing and revision of the data presented.

Therefore, this handy carbohydrate counter will provide each year the most current and accurate estimates available. Generous use of this little book will help you and your family to select the right foods and the proper number of carbohydrates each member requires.

Good eating in 1984! For 1985, we'll pick up the new products, drop any has-beens, and make whatever other changes are necessary.

Barbara Kraus

Why This Book?

Some of the data presented here can be found in more detail in my best-selling *Calories and Carbohydrates,* a dictionary of 8,000 brand names and basic foods. Complete as it is, it is meant to be used as a reference book at home or in the office and not to be squeezed into a suit jacket or evening bag—it's just too big.

Therefore, responding to the need for a portable carbohydrate guide, and one which can reflect food changes often, I have written this smaller and handier version. The selection of material and the additional new entries provide readers with pertinent data on thousands of products that they would prepare at home to take to work, eat in a restaurant or luncheonette, nibble on from the coffee cart, take to the beach, buy in the candy store, etcetera.

For the sake of saving space and providing you with a greater selection of products, I had to make certain compromises: whereas in the giant book there are several physical descriptions of a product, here there is but one.

What Are Carbohydrates?

Carbohydrates—which include sugars, starches, and acids—are one of several chemical compounds in food which yield calories. Their main function is to supply energy to body cells, particularly muscle and brain cells. The amount of carbohydrates varies from zero in meats, fish, and poultry, to heavy concentrations in such foods as syrups, cereals, bread, beans, some fresh and all dried fruit, and root vegetables, such as potatoes.

As of this date, the most respected nutritional researchers insist that some carbohydrate is necessary every day for maintaining good health. The amount to be included is an individual matter, and in any drastic effort to alter your eating patterns, be sure to consult your doctor first.

ABBREVIATIONS AND SYMBOLS

* = prepared as package directs[1]
< = less than
& = and
" = inch
canned = bottles or jars as well as cans
dia. = diameter
fl. = fluid
liq. = liquid
lb. = pound
med. = medium

oz. = ounce
pkg. = package
pt. = pint
qt. = quart
sq. = square
T. = tablespoon
Tr. = trace
tsp. = teaspoon
wt. = weight

Italics or name in parentheses = registered trademark, ®. All data not identified by company or trademark are based on material obtained from the United States Department of Agriculture or Health, Education and Welfare/Food and Agriculture Organization.

EQUIVALENTS

By Weight	By Volume
1 pound = 16 ounces	1 quart = 4 cups
1 ounce = 28.35 grams	1 cup = 8 fluid ounces
3.52 ounces = 100 grams	1 cup = ½ pint
	1 cup = 16 tablespoons
	2 tablespoons = 1 fluid ounce
	1 tablespoon = 3 teaspoons
	1 pound butter = 4 sticks or 2 cups

[1]If the package directions call for whole or skim milk, the data given here are for whole milk unless otherwise stated.

Food and Description	Measure or Quantity	Carbohydrates (grams)

A

Food and Description	Measure or Quantity	Carbohydrates (grams)
ABALONE, canned	4 oz.	2.6
AC'CENT	¼ tsp.	
ACEROLA, fresh, fruit	4 oz.	7.7
ALEXANDER COCKTAIL MIX, (Holland House)	1 serving	16.0
ALLSPICE (French's)	1 tsp.	1.3
ALMOND:		
In shell	10 nuts	2.0
Shelled, raw, natural with skins	1 oz.	5.5
Roasted, dry (Planters)	1 oz.	6.0
Roasted, oil (Fisher)	1 oz.	5.5
ALPHA-BITS, cereal (Post)	1 cup (1 oz.)	24.6
AMARETTO DI SARONNO	1 fl. oz.	9.0
A.M. FRUIT DRINK (Mott's)	6 fl. oz.	22.0
ANCHOVY, PICKLED, canned, flat or rolled, not heavily salted, drained	2-oz. can	.1
ANISE SEED, dried	½ oz.	6.3
ANISETTE:		
(DeKuyper)	1 fl. oz.	11.4
(Mr. Boston)	1 fl. oz.	10.8
APPLE:		
Eaten with skin	2½" dia.	15.3
Eaten without skin	2½" dia.	13.9
Canned (Comstock):		
Rings, drained	1 ring	7.0
Sliced	⅙ of 21-oz. can	10.0
Dried:		
(Del Monte)	1 cup	37.2
(Sun Maid)	2-oz. serving	40.0
Frozen, sweetened	10-oz. pkg.	68.9
APPLE BROWN BETTY	1 cup	63.9
APPLE BUTTER (Smucker's) cider	1 T.	9.0
APPLE-CHERRY JUICE; COCKTAIL, canned *Musselman's*	8 fl. oz.	28.0
APPLE CIDER:		
Canned (Mott's) sweet	½ cup	14.6
*Mix, *Country Time**	8 fl. oz.	24.5
APPLE-CRANBERRY DRINK (Hi-C)		
Canned	6 fl. oz.	21.0
*Mix	6 fl. oz.	18.0

Food and Description	Measure or Quantity	Carbohydrates (grams)
APPLE-CRANBERRY JUICE,		
canned (Lincoln)	6 fl. oz.	25.0
APPLE DRINK:		
Canned:		
Capri Sun, natural	6¾ fl. oz.	22.7
(Hi-C)	6 fl. oz.	23.0
*Mix (Hi-C)	6 fl. oz.	18.0
APPLE DUMPLINGS, frozen		
(Pepperidge Farm)	1 dumpling	33.0
APPLE, ESCALLOPED, frozen		
(Stouffer's)	4 oz.	27.8
APPLE-GRAPE JUICE, canned:		
Musselman's	6 fl. oz.	21.0
(Red Cheek)	6 fl. oz.	22.6
APPLE JACKS, cereal (Kellogg's)	1 cup (1 oz.)	26.0
APPLE JAM (Smucker's)	1 T.	13.5
APPLE JELLY:		
Sweetened (Smucker's)	1 T.	14.0
Dietetic (See APPLE SPREAD)		
APPLE JUICE:		
Canned:		
(Lincoln)	6 fl. oz.	24.0
(Minute Maid)	6 fl. oz.	24.0
(Mott's)	6 fl. oz.	19.0
Musselman's	6 fl. oz.	21.0
(Red Cheek)	6 fl. oz.	21.2
(Seneca Foods)	6 fl. oz.	22.0
Chilled (Minute Maid)	6 fl. oz.	24.0
*Frozen:		
(Minute Maid)	6 fl. oz.	24.0
(Seneca Foods) Vitamin C added	6 fl. oz.	22.0
(Seneca Foods) natural style,		
Vitamin C added	6 fl. oz.	22.0
APPLE PIE (See PIE, Apple)		
APPLE SAUCE:		
Regular:		
(Del Monte)	½ cup	23.6
(Mott's):		
Natural	½ cup	27.5
With ground cranberries	½ cup	27.0
Musselman's	½ cup	23.5
(Stokely-Van Camp)	½ cup	22.5
Dietetic:		
(Diet Delight)	½ cup	13.0
(Featherweight) water pack	½ cup	12.0
(Mott's) natural	4-oz. serving	11.0

Food and Description	Measure or Quantity	Carbohydrates (grams)
Musselman's, natural	½ cup	12.0
(S&W) *Nutradiet*	½ cup	14.0
APPLE SPREAD, low sugar:		
(Dia-Mel)	1 T	0.
(Diet Delight)	1 T	3.0
(Featherweight):		
Regular	1 T	4.0
Artificially sweetened	1 T	1.0
(Tillie Lewis) *Tasti Diet*	1 T	3.0
APPLE STRUDEL, frozen		
(Pepperidge Farm)	3-oz. serving	35.0
APRICOT:		
Fresh, whole	1 apricot	4.5
Canned, regular pack:		
(Del Monte)		
whole, peeled	1 cup	53.2
(Libby's) halves, heavy syrup	1 cup	53.6
(Stokely-Van Camp)	1 cup	54.0
Canned, dietetic:		
(Del Monte) *Lite*	½ cup	15.1
(Diet Delight):		
Syrup pack	½ cup	15.0
Water pack	½ cup	9.0
(Featherweight):		
Juice pack	½ cup	12.0
Water pack	½ cup	9.0
(Libby's) Lite	½ cup	15.0
(S&W) *Nutradiet:*		
Halves, juice pack	½ cup	13.0
Halves, water pack	½ cup	9.0
Whole, juice pack	½ cup	10.0
Dried:		
(Del Monte)	2-oz. serving	37.8
(Sun-Maid; Sunsweet)	¼ cup (1.7 oz.)	30.0
APRICOT LIQUEUR (DeKuyper)	1 fl. oz.	8.3
APRICOT NECTAR:		
(Del Monte)	6 fl. oz.	27.0
(Libby's)	6 fl. oz.	27.0
APRICOT-PINEAPPLE NECTAR, canned, dietetic (S&W) *Nutradiet*	6-oz. serving	12.0
APRICOT & PINEAPPLE PRESERVE OR JAM:		
Sweetened (Smucker's)	1 T.	13.5
Dietetic (See APRICOT & PINEAPPLE SPREAD)		

Food and Description	Measure or Quantity	Carbohydrates (grams)
APRICOT & PINEAPPLE SPREAD,		
low sugar:		
(Diet Delight)	1 T.	3.0
(Featherweight) artificially sweetened	1 T.	1.0
(S&W) *Nutradiet*	1 T.	3.0
(Tillie Lewis) *Tasti Diet*	1 T.	3.0
APRICOT SOUR COCKTAIL		
(National Distillers-*Duet*)		
12½% alcohol	2 fl. oz.	1.6
ARBY'S:		
Beef and Cheese sandwich	6 oz.	36.0
Club sandwich	9 oz.	43.0
Ham'n Cheese	5½ oz.	33.0
Roast Beef:		
Reguar	5 oz.	32.0
Junior	3 oz.	21.0
Super	9¾ oz.	61.0
Turkey Deluxe	8½ oz.	46.0
ARTICHOKE:		
Boiled	15-oz. artichoke	42.1
Canned (Cara Mia) marinated, drained	6-oz. jar	12.6
Frozen:		
(Birds Eye) deluxe, hearts	⅓ pkg.	6.6
(Cara Mia)	3-oz. serving	7.5
ASPARAGUS:		
Boiled	1 spear (½" dia. at base)	.5
Canned, regular pack, spears, solids & liq.:		
(Del Monte) green or white	1 cup	6.8
(Green Giant) green	8-oz. can	6.4
Musselman's	1 cup	6.0
(Stokely-Van Camp)	1 cup	6.0
Canned, dietetic, solids & liq.:		
(Diet Delight)	½ cup	2.0
(Featherweight) cut spears	1 cup	6.0
(S&W) *Nutradiet*	1 cup	8.0
Frozen:		
(Birds Eye):		
Cuts	⅓ pkg.	3.8
Spears, regular or jumbo deluxe	⅓ pkg.	3.9
(Green Giant) cuts, butter sauce	3 oz.	4.6
(McKenzie)	⅓ pkg.	4.0
(Seabrook Farms)	⅓ pkg.	3.8
(Stouffer's) souffle	⅓ pkg.	8.0

Food and Description	Measure or Quantity	Carbohydrates (grams)
AUNT JEMIMA SYRUP (See SYRUP)		
AVOCADO, all varieties	1 fruit	14.3
***AWAKE** (Birds Eye)	6 fl. oz.	21.9
AYDS, butterscotch	1 piece	5.7

B

BACON, broiled (Oscar Mayer):		
Regular slice	6-gram slice	.1
Thick slice	1 slice	.2
BACON BITS:		
(Betty Crocker) *Bac*Os*	1 tsp.	.6
(Durkee) imitation	1 tsp.	.5
(French's) imitation	1 tsp.	Tr.
(Libby's) crumbles	1 tsp.	.7
(Oscar Mayer) real	1 tsp.	.1
BACON, CANADIAN, unheated:		
(Hormel) sliced	1-oz. serving	.1
(Oscar Mayer) 93% fat free	.7-oz. slice	0.
(Oscar Mayer) 93% fat free	1-oz. slice	0.
BACON, SIMULATED, cooked:		
(Oscar Mayer) *Lean 'N Tasty:*		
Beef	1 slice	.2
Pork	1 slice	.2
(Swift) *Sizzlean*	1 strip	0.
BAGEL:		
Egg	3-inch diameter, 1.9 oz.	28.3
Water	3-inch diameter, 1.9 oz.	30.5
BAKING POWDER, (Featherweight) low sodium, cereal free	1 tsp.	2.0
BAMBOO SHOOTS:		
Raw, trimmed	¼ lb.	5.9
Canned, drained:		
(Chun King)	½ of 8½-oz. can	3.0
(La Choy)	½ cup	2.2
BANANA, medium (weighed unpeeled)	6.3-oz. banana	26.4
BARBECUE SEASONING (French's)	1 tsp.	1.0
BARDOLINO WINE (Antinori)	1 fl. oz.	6.3
BARLEY, pearled (Quaker Scotch)	¼ cup	36.3
BASIL (French's)	1 tsp.	.7

5

Food and Description	Measure or Quantity	Carbohydrates (grams)
BASS:		
Baked, stuffed	3½″ × 4½″ × 1½″	23.4
Oven-fried	8¾″ × 4½″ × ⅝″	13.4
BAY LEAF (French's)	1 tsp.	1.0
B & B LIQUEUR	1 fl. oz.	5.7
B.B.Q. Sauce & Beef, frozen		
(Banquet) *Cookin' Bag*, sliced	5-oz. cooking bag	12.5
BEAN, BAKED:		
(USDA):		
With pork & molasses sauce	1 cup	53.8
With pork & tomato sauce	1 cup	48.5
Canned:		
(B&M):		
Pea bean with pork in brown sugar sauce	8 oz.	49.0
Red kidney bean in brown sugar sauce	8 oz.	50.0
(Campbell):		
Home style	8-oz. can	48.0
With pork & tomato sauce	8-oz. can	49.0
(Grandma Brown's)	8-oz. serving	54.1
(Libby's):		
Deep Brown, with pork & molasses sauce	½ of 14-oz. can	40.6
Deep Brown, vegetarian in tomato sauce	½ of 14-oz. can	40.8
(Sultana) with pork & tomato sauce	½ of 16-oz. can	41.8
(Van Camp) with pork	8 oz.	41.3
BEAN, BARBECUE (Campbell)	7⅞-oz. can	43.0
BEAN, BLACK, DRY	1 cup	122.4
BEAN, BROWN, DRY	1 cup	122.4
BEAN & FRANKFURTER, canned:		
(Campbell) in tomato and molasses sauce	8-oz. can	42.0
(Hormel) *Short Orders*, 'n weiners	7½-oz. can	29.0
BEAN & FRANKFURTER DINNER, frozen:		
(Banquet)	10¾-oz. dinner	63.1
(Swanson) *TV Brand*	11¼-oz. dinner	62.0
BEAN, GARBANZO, canned, dietetic (S&W) *Nutradiet*, low sodium	½ cup	19.0
BEAN, GREEN:		
Boiled, 1½″ to 2″ pieces, drained	½ cup	3.7
Canned, regular pack:		
(Comstock) solids & liq.	½ cup	4.0
(Del Monte) French, drained,	½ cup	4.9

Food and Description	Measure or Quantity	Carbohydrates (grams)
(Green Giant) French or whole, solids & liq.	½ of 8½-oz. can	4.2
(Libby's) French, solids & liq.	½ cup	4.0
(Stokely-Van Camp) solids & liq.	½ cup	4.0
(Sunshine) solids & liq.	½ cup	3.8
Canned, dietetic:		
(Diet Delight) solids & liq.	½ cup	3.0
(Featherweight) cut or French, solids & liq.	½ cup	5.0
(S&W) *Nutradiet*, cut, solids & liq., low sodium	½ cup	4.0
Frozen:		
(Birds Eye):		
Cut	⅓ pkg.	5.9
French, with mushrooms	⅓ pkg.	6.5
Italian style	⅓ pgk.	7.3
Whole, deluxe	⅓ pkg.	5.1
(Green Giant):		
With butter sauce	⅓ pkg.	4.8
With mushroom in cream sauce	⅓ pkg.	7.9
(McKenzie) cut or French style	⅓ pkg.	6.0
(Seabrook Farms)	⅓ pkg.	5.8
(Southland) cut or French style	⅓ of 16-oz. pkg.	5.0
BEAN, GREEN, & MUSHROOM CASSEROLE (Stouffer's)	½ pkg.	11.9
BEAN, GREEN, WITH POTATOES, canned (Sunshine) solids & liq.	½ cup	7.0
BEAN, GREEN, PUREE, canned, dietetic (Featherweight)	1 cup	15.0
BEAN, ITALIAN:		
Canned (Del Monte) drained	½ cup	8.2
Frozen (McKenzie; Seabrook Farms)	⅓ pkg.	7.1
BEAN, KIDNEY:		
Canned, regular pack:		
(Furman) red, fancy, light	½ cup	21.2
(Van Camp):		
Light	8 oz.	35.9
New Orleans style	8 oz.	33.8
Red	8 oz.	37.9
Canned, dietetic (S&W) *Nutradiet*, low sodium, solids & liq.	½ cup	16.0
BEAN, LIMA:		
Boiled, drained	½ cup	16.8
Canned, regular pack:		
(Del Monte) drained	½ cup	19.6

7

Food and Description	Measure or Quantity	Carbohydrates (grams)
(Libby's) solids & liq.	½ cup	16.0
(Sultana) butter bean	¼ of 15-oz. can	14.6
Canned, dietetic		
(Featherweight) solids & liq.	½ cup	16.0
Frozen:		
(Birds Eye) tiny, deluxe	⅓ pkg.	20.3
(Green Giant):		
In butter sauce	3 oz.	15.5
Harvest Fresh	4 oz.	21.8
(McKenzie):		
Baby lima	⅓ pkg.	24.0
Fordhook	⅓ pkg.	19.0
Tiny	⅓ pgk.	21.0
(Seabrook Farms):		
Baby lima	⅓ pkg.	23.6
Baby butter bean	⅓ pkg.	26.1
Fordhooks	⅓ pkg.	17.9
BEAN, PINTO (Del Monte) spicy	½ cup	19.0
BEAN, REFRIED, canned:		
(Del Monte) regular or spicy	½ cup	20.0
Old El Paso	½ of 8¼-oz. can	17.5
(Ortega) lightly spicy or true bean	½ cup	25.0
BEAN, SALAD, canned		
(Green Giant)	4¼-oz. serving	18.5
BEAN SOUP (*See* SOUP, Bean)		
BEAN SPROUT:		
Mung, raw	½ lb.	15.0
Mung, boiled, drained	¼ lb.	5.9
Soy, raw	½ lb.	12.0
Soy, boiled, drained	¼ lb.	4.2
Canned:		
(Chun King) drained	8 oz.	2.0
(La Choy) drained	⅔ cup	.9
BEAN, YELLOW OR WAX:		
Boiled, 1″ pieces, drained	½ cup	2.9
Canned, regular pack:		
(Comstock) solids & liqs.	½ cup	4.5
(Del Monte) cut, solids & liqs.	½ cup	3.4
(Festal) cut or French style, solids & liq.	½ cups	3.6
(Libby's) cut, solids & liqs.	4 oz.	4.0
(Stokely-Van Camp) solids & liq.	½ cup	4.4
Canned, dietetic (Featherweight, cut, solids & liq.)	½ cup	5.0
Frozen (McKenzie) cut	⅓ pkg.	5.0
BEEF	Any quantity	0.

Food and Description	Measure or Quantity	Carbohydrates (grams)
BEEFAMATO COCKTAIL (Mott's)	6 fl. oz.	15.0
BEEF BOUILLON:		
(Herb-Ox):		
Cube	1 cube	.7
Packet	1 packet	.9
MBT	1 packet	2.0
Low sodium (Featherweight)	1 tsp.	2.0
BEEF, CHIPPED:		
Frozen:		
(Banquet) creamed, *Cookin' Bag*	5-oz. pkg.	10.5
(Stouffer's) creamed	5½-oz.	10.0
(Swanson) creamed	10½-oz. entree	16.0
BEEF DINNER or ENTREE, frozen:		
(Banquet):		
Regular	11-oz. dinner	20.9
Chopped	11-oz. dinner	32.8
Man Pleaser, sliced	20-oz. dinner	63.7
(Morton):		
Regular	10-oz. dinner	20.0
Country Table, sliced	14-oz. dinner	55.7
Steak House, sirloin strip	9½-oz. dinner	43.2
(Swanson):		
Hungry Man, chopped	18-oz. dinner	50.0
Hungry Man, sliced	12¼-oz. dinner	20.0
TV Brand, chopped sirloin	10-oz. dinner	33.0
3-course	15-oz. dinner	50.0
(Weight-Watchers):		
Beefsteak, 2-compartment meal	9¾-oz. pkg.	12.0
Sirloin in mushroom sauce, 3-compartment meal	13-oz. pkg.	16.0
BEEF, GROUND, SEASONING MIX:		
*(Durkee):		
Regular	1 cup	9.0
With onion	1 cup	6.5
(French's) with onion	1⅛-oz. pkg.	24.0
BEEF, HASH, ROAST:		
Canned, *Mary Kitchen:*		
Regular	7½-oz. serving	17.9
Short Orders	7½-oz. can	19.0
Frozen (Stouffer's)	½ of 11½-oz. serving	10.9
BEEF PEPPER ORIENTAL:		
*Canned (La Choy):		
Regular	¾ cup	12.0
Bi-pack	¾ cup	8.0

Food and Description	Measure or Quantity	Carbohydrates (grams)
Frozen (Chun King):		
Dinner	11-oz. dinner	43.0
Pouch	6-oz. serving	10.0
BEEF PIE, frozen:		
(Banquet):		
Regular	8-oz. pie	40.9
Supreme	8-oz. pie	38.0
(Stouffer's)	10-oz. pie	37.8
(Swanson):		
Regular	8-oz. pie	40.0
Hungry-Man	16-oz. pie	65.0
BEEF PUFFS, frozen (Durkee)	1 piece	3.0
BEEF, SHORT RIBS, frozen (Stouffer's) boneless, with vegetable gravy	½ of 11½-oz. pkg.	2.0
BEEF SOUP (See SOUP, Beef)		
BEEF SPREAD, ROAST, canned (Underwood)	½ of 4¾-oz. can	Tr.
BEEF STEW:		
Home recipe, made with lean beef chuck	1 cup	15.2
Canned, regular pack:		
Dinty Moore:		
Regular	7½-oz. serving	12.8
Short Orders	7½-oz. can	14.0
(Libby's)	8-oz.	19.0
(Swanson)	7⅝-oz. serving	16.0
Canned, dietetic (Featherweight)	7½-oz.	24.0
Frozen:		
(Banquet) *Buffet Supper*	2-lb. pkg.	90.9
(Green Giant):		
Boil 'N Bag	9-oz. entree	19.7
Twin Pouch, with noodles	9-oz. entree	34.5
(Stouffer's)	10-oz. serving	15.9
BEEF STEW SEASONING MIX:		
*(Durkee)	1 cup	16.7
(French's)	1 pkg.	30.0
BEEF STOCK BASE (French's)	1 tsp.	2.0
BEEF STIX (Vienna)	1 oz.	1.4
BEEF STROGANOFF, frozen (Stouffer's) with parsley noodles	9¾ oz.	30.7
***BEEF STROGANOFF SEASONING MIX** (DURKEE)	1 cup	71.2
BEER & ALE:		
Regular:		
Black Horse Ale	8 fl. oz.	8.9

Food and Description	Measure or Quantity	Carbohydrates (grams)
Budweiser	8 fl. oz.	8.8
Michelob	8 fl. oz.	9.0
Schmidt, 3.2 low gravity	8 fl. oz.	11.9
Light or low carbohydrate:		
Budweiser Light	8 fl. oz.	3.8
Michelob, light	8 fl. oz.	7.8
Natural Light	8 fl. oz.	4.0
Stroh Light	8 fl. oz.	4.7
BEER, NEAR:		
Goetz Pale	8 fl. oz.	2.6
Kingsbury (Heileman)	8 fl. oz.	7.1
BEET:		
Boiled, whole	2″ dia. beet	3.6
Boiled, sliced	½ cup	7.3
Canned, regular pack:		
(Del Monte):		
Pickled, solids & liq.	½ cup	18.0
Sliced, drained	½ cup	7.6
(Greenwood):		
Harvard, solids & liq.	½ cup	16.0
Pickled, solids & liq.	½ cup	27.5
Pickled, with onion, solids & liq.	½ cup	27.5
(Libby's) Harvard, solids & liq.	½ cup	20.8
(Stokely-Van Camp) pickled,		
solids & liq.	½ cup	22.5
Canned, dietetic:		
(Blue Boy) whole, solids & liq.	½ cup	9.2
(Comstock) solids & liq.	½ cup	6.5
(Featherweight) sliced, solids & liq.	½ cup	10.0
(S&W) *Nutradiet*, sliced, solids & liq.	½ cup	9.0
BEET PUREE, canned, dietetic (Featherweight)	1 cup	20.0
BENEDICTINE LIQUEUR		
(Julius Wile)	1½ fl. oz.	10.3
BIG H, burger sauce (Hellmann's)	1 T.	1.6
BIG MAC (See McDonald's)		
BIG WHEEL (Hostess)	1 cake	21.5
BISCUIT DOUGH (Pillsbury):		
Baking Powder, *1869 Brand*	1 biscuit	13.5
Big Country	1 biscuit	15.5
Big Country, Good 'N Buttery	1 biscuit	14.0
Buttermilk:		
Regular	1 biscuit	10.0
Extra Lights	1 biscuit	10.5
Flaky, *Hungry Jack*	1 biscuit	13.0

Food and Description	Measure or Quantity	Carbohydrates (grams)
Butter Tastin', 1869 Brand	1 biscuit	11.0
Butter Tastin', Hungry Jack	1 biscuit	12.0
Dinner	1 biscuit	7.5
Oven Ready, Ballard	1 biscuit	9.5
BITTERS (Angostura)	1 tsp.	2.1
BLACKBERRY JELLY:		
Sweetened (Smucker's)	1 T.	13.5
Dietetic (See Blackberry Spread)		
BLACKBERRY LIQUEUR (Bols)	1 fl. oz.	8.9
BLACKBERRY PRESERVE OR JAM:		
Sweetened (Smucker's)	1 T.	13.5
Dietetic:		
(Dia-Mel)	1 T.	Tr.
(Diet-Delight)	1 T.	3.3
(Featherweight)	1 T.	4.0
(S&W) *Nutradiet*	1 T.	3.0
BLACKBERRY SPREAD, low sugar:		
(Diet Delight)	1 T.	3.0
(Featherweight)	1 T.	4.0
(Smucker's)	1 T.	6.0
BLACKBERRY WINE		
(Mogen David)	3 fl. oz.	18.7
BLACK-EYED PEAS:		
Canned:		
(Sultana) with pork	7½-oz. serving	33.9
(Sunshine) with pork, solids & liq.	½ cup	16.1
Frozen:		
(McKenzie)	⅓ pkg.	23.0
(Seabrook Farms)	⅓ pkg.	22.7
(Southland)	⅓ of 16-oz. pkg.	21.0
BLINTZE, frozen (King Kold) cheese	2½-oz. piece	21.4
BLOODY MARY MIX:		
Dry (Bar-Tender's)	1 serving	5.7
Liquid (Sacramento)	5½-fl.-oz. can	9.1
BLUEBERRY, fresh, whole	½ lb.	31.9
BLUEBERRY PIE		
(*See* PIE, Blueberry)		
BLUEBERRY PRESERVE OR JAM:		
Sweetened (Smucker's)	1 T.	13.5
Dietetic (Dia-Mel)	1 T.	0.
BLUEFISH, broiled	3½″ × 3″ × ½″ piece	0.

12

Food and Description	Measure or Quantity	Carbohydrates (grams)
BODY BUDDIES, cereal (General Mills):		
Brown sugar & honey	1 cup	24.0
Natural fruit flavor	¾ cup	24.0
BOLOGNA:		
(Best's Kosher):		
Chub	1-oz. serving	1.0
Sliced	1-oz. serving	1.0
(Eckrich):		
Beef, garlic, pickled, ring or sliced	1 oz.	1.5
Thick sliced	1.7-oz. slice	3.0
(Hormel):		
Beef	1-oz. slice	.3
Fine ground, ring	1-oz. serving	.6
Meat	1-oz. slice	.2
(Oscar Mayer):		
Beef	.8-oz. slice	.6
Beef	1-oz. slice	.8
Beef	1.3-oz. slice	1.1
Meat	.8-oz. slice	.4
Meat	1-oz. slice	.5
(Swift)	1-oz. slice	1.5
(Vienna) beef	1-oz. serving	.7
BOLOGNA & CHEESE		
(Oscar Mayer)	.8-oz. slice	.6
BONITO, canned (Star-Kist)	Any quantity	0.
BOO*BERRY cereal (General Mills)	1 cup	24.0
BORSCHT, canned:		
Regular:		
(Gold's)	8-oz. serving	17.5
(Mother's) old fashioned	8-oz. serving	21.3
Dietetic or low calorie:		
(Gold's)	8-oz. serving	17.5
(Mother's):		
Artificially sweetened	8-oz. serving	6.1
Unsalted	8-oz. serving	25.1
(Rokeach)	8-oz. serving	6.7
BOSCO (See SYRUP)		
*BOWL O'NOODLES		
(Nestlé), beef or chicken	1½-oz. envelope	29.0
BOYSENBERRY JELLY:		
Sweetened (Smucker's)	1 T.	13.5
Dietetic (See Boysenberry Spread)		
BOYSENBERRY SPREAD,		
(Smucker's)		
low sugar	1 T.	6.0

Food and Description	Measure or Quantity	Carbohydrates (grams)
(S&W) *Nutradiet*	1 T.	3.0
BRAN, crude	1 oz.	17.5
BRAN, Miller's	1 oz.	13.7
BRAN BREAKFAST CEREAL:		
(Crawford's) & dates	⅓ cup	20.0
(Kellogg's):		
All Bran or *Bran Buds*	⅓ cup	22.0
Cracklin' Bran	½ cup	20.0
40% bran flakes	¾ cup	23.0
Raisin	¾ cup	30.0
(Nabisco)	½ cup	21.0
(Post) 40% bran flakes	⅔ cup	22.5
(Quaker) *Corn Bran*	⅔ cup	23.3
(Ralston-Purina):		
Bran Chex	⅔ cup	23.0
40% bran	¾ cup	23.0
Raisin	¾ cup	30.0
BRANDY, FLAVORED		
(Mr. Boston):		
Apricot	1 fl. oz.	8.9
Blackberry	1 fl. oz.	8.6
Cherry	1 fl. oz.	7.4
Coffee	1 fl. oz.	10.6
Ginger	1 fl. oz.	3.5
Peach	1 fl. oz.	8.9
BRAUNSCHWEIGER:		
(Oscar Mayer) chub	1 oz.	.7
(Swift) 8-oz. chub	1 oz.	1.4
BRAZIL NUT, roasted (Fisher)		
salted	1-oz. serving	3.1
BREAD:		
Apple (Pepperidge Farm)	.9-oz. slice	13.0
Cinnamon (Pepperidge Farm)	.9-oz. slice	12.5
Corn & molasses (Pepperidge Farm)	.9-oz. slice	15.0
Cracked wheat (Wonder)	1-oz. slice	13.6
Crispbread, *Wasa:*		
Mora	3.2-oz. slice	70.5
Rye, golden	.4-oz. slice	7.8
Rye, lite	.3-oz. slice	6.2
Sesame	.5-oz. slice	10.6
Sport	.4-oz. slice	9.1
Date nut roll (Dromedary)	1-oz. slice	13.0
Date walnut (Pepperidge Farm)	.9-oz. slice	11.5
Flatbread, *Ideal:*		
Bran	.2-oz. slice	4.1
Extra thin	.1-oz. slice	2.5

Food and Description	Measure or Quantity	Carbohydrates (grams)
Whole grain	.2-oz. slice	4.0
French:		
(Pepperidge Farm)	2-oz. slice	28.0
(Wonder)	1-oz. slice	13.6
Hillbilly	1-oz. slice	13.6
Hollywood, dark	1-oz. slice	12.5
Honey bran (Pepperidge Farm)	1 slice	13.0
Honey, wheat berry (Arnold)	1.2-oz. slice	16.0
Italian (Pepperidge Farm)	2-oz. slice	27.0
Low Sodium (Wonder)	1-oz. slice	13.6
Oatmeal (Pepperidge Farm)	1 slice	12.5
Protogen Protein (Thomas')	.7-oz. slice	7.4
Pumpernickel:		
(Arnold)	1-oz. slice	14.0
(Levy's)	1-oz. slice	15.5
(Pepperidge Farm):		
Regular	1 slice	15.5
Party	1 slice	3.0
Raisin:		
(Arnold) tea	.9-oz. slice	13.0
(Pepperidge Farm) with cinnamon	.9-oz. slice	14.0
(Sun-Maid)	1-oz. slice	14.5
(Thomas') cinnamon	.8-oz. slice	11.7
Roman Meal	1-oz. slice	13.6
Rye:		
(Arnold) Jewish	1.1-oz. slice	14.0
(Levy's) real	1-oz. slice	15.0
(Pepperidge Farm) family	1 slice	15.5
(Wonder)	1-oz. slice	12.8
Sahara (Thomas'):		
Wheat	1-oz. piece	13.7
White	1-oz. piece	16.0
Sour dough, *Di Carlo*	1-oz. slice	13.6
Sprouted wheat (Pepperidge Farm)	.9-oz. slice	11.5
Vienna (Pepperidge Farm)	.9-oz. slice	13.5
Wheat:		
Fresh Horizons	1-oz. slice	9.6
Fresh & Natural	1-oz. slice	13.6
Home Pride	1-oz. slice	13.1
(Pepperidge Farm) family	.9-oz. slice	13.0
(Wonder) regular	1-oz. slice	13.6
Wheatberry, *Home Pride*	1-oz. slice	13.3
Wheat Germ (Pepperidge Farm)	1 slice	12.5
White:		
(Arnold):		
Brick Oven	.8-oz. slice	11.0

Food and Description	Measure or Quantity	Carbohydrates (grams)
Country	1.2-oz. slice	17.0
Measure Up	.5-oz. slice	7.0
Home pride	1-oz. slice	13.1
(Pepperidge Farm):		
Large loaf	.9-oz. slice	13.5
Sandwich	.8-oz. slice	11.5
Sliced, 1-lb. loaf	.9-oz. slice	13.0
Toasting	1.2-oz. slice	16.0
(Wonder) regular or buttermilk	1-oz. slice	13.4
Whole wheat:		
(Arnold) *Brick Oven*	.8-oz. slice	9.5
(Arnold) *Measure Up*	.5-oz. slice	6.5
(Pepperidge Farm) thin slice	1 slice	12.0
(Thomas') 100%	.8-oz. slice	10.1
(Wonder) 100%	1-oz. slice	11.9
BREAD, CANNED,		
brown, plain or raisin (B&M)	½" slice	18.0
BREAD, CRUMBS (Contadina)		
seasoned	½ cup	40.6
BREAD DOUGH, frozen:		
(Pepperidge Farm):		
Country Rye	⅒ of loaf	13.5
White	⅒ of loaf	14.0
(Rich's):		
French or Italian	¹⁄₂₀ of loaf	11.0
Raisin	¹⁄₂₀ of loaf	12.3
Wheat	.5-oz. slice	10.5
White	.8-oz. slice	9.4
***BREAD MIX** (Pillsbury):*		
Applesauce spice	¹⁄₁₂ of loaf	28.0
Apricot nut, banana or carrot nut	¹⁄₁₂ of loaf	27.0
Blueberry nut	¹⁄₁₂ of loaf	26.0
Cherry nut or cranberry	¹⁄₁₂ of loaf	30.0
Date or nut	¹⁄₁₂ of loaf	31.0
BREAKFAST BAR (Carnation):		
Almond crunch	1 piece	20.0
All other varieties	1 piece	22.0
BREAKFAST DRINK,		
(Pillsbury)	1 pouch	38.0
BREAKFAST SQUARES (General		
Mills) all flavors	1 bar	22.5
BRIGHT & EARLY	6 fl. oz.	21.6
BROCCOLI:		
Boiled, whole stalk	1 stalk	19.0
Boiled, ½" pieces	½ cup	16.0

Food and Description	Measure or Quantity	Carbohydrates (grams)
Frozen:		
(Birds Eye) in cheese sauce	⅓ pkg.	7.9
(Birds Eye) in Hollandaise sauce	⅓ pkg.	4.1
(Green Giant)		
spears in butter sauce	⅓ pkg	5.3
(Green Giant):		
in cheese sauce	3⅓ oz.	6.8
cuts, polybag	½ cup	2.7
(McKenzie) chopped or spears	⅓ pkg.	5.0
(Mrs. Paul's) in cheese sauce	⅓ pkg.	18.8
(Seabrook Farms) chopped or		
spears	⅓ pk	4.1
(Stouffer's) au gratin	⅓ pkg.	4.6
BRUSSELS SPROUT:		
Boiled	3–4 sprouts	4.9
Frozen:		
(Birds Eye) baby with cheese sauce	⅓ pkg.	9.3
(Birds Eye) baby	⅓ pkg.	7.3
(Green Giant)		
in butter sauce	⅓ pkg	8.2
(Green Giant) halves in cheese		
sauce	⅓ pkg.	10.8
(Stouffer's) au gratin	⅓ pkg.	10.6
BUCKWHEAT, cracked (Pocono)	1 oz.	19.4
BUC*WHEATS, cereal (General		
Mills)	1 oz. (¾ cup)	24.0
BULGUR, canned, seasoned	4-oz. serving	37.2
BULLWINKLE PUDDING STIX,		
Good Humor	2½-fl. oz. bar	20.0
BURGER KING:		
Apple pie	3-oz. pie	32.0
Cheeseburger	1 burger	30.0
Cheeseburger, double meat	1 burger	32.0
Coca Cola	1 medium sized drink	31.0
French fries	1 regular order	25.0
Hamburger	1 burger	29.0
Onion rings	1 regular order	29.0
Pepsi, diet	1 medium-sized drink	1.0
Shake, chocolate or vanilla	1 shake	57.0
Whopper:		
Regular	1 burger	50.0
Regular, with cheese	1 burger	52.0
Double beef	1 burger	52.0
Double beef, with cheese	1 burger	54.0

17

Food and Description	Measure or Quantity	Carbohydrates (grams)
Junior	1 burger	31.0
Junior, with cheese	1 burger	32.0
BURGUNDY WINE:		
(Great Western)	3 fl. oz.	2.3
(Louis M. Martini)	3 fl. oz.	.2
(Paul Masson)	3 fl. oz.	2.2
(Taylor)	3 fl. oz.	3.3
BURGUNDY WINE, SPARKLING:		
(B&G)	3 fl. oz.	2.2
(Taylor)	3 fl. oz.	4.2
BURRITO:		
*Canned (Del Monte)	1 burrito	39.0
Frozen:		
(Hormel):		
Beef	1 burrito	28.4
Cheese	1 burrito	32.7
Hot chili	1 burrito	32.0
(Van de Kamp's) & guacamole		
sauce	½ of 12-oz. pkg.	40.0
BURRITO FILLING MIX, canned		
(Del Monte)	1 cup	39.0
BUTTER:		
Regular (Breakstone)	1 T.	<1
Regular (Meadow Gold)	1 tsp.	0.
Whipped (Breakstone)	1 T.	<1
BUTTERSCOTCH MORSELS		
(Nestlé)	1 oz.	19.0

C

CABBAGE:		
Boiled, without salt, until tender	½ cup (2.6 oz.)	3.1
Canned:		
(Comstock) red, solids & liq.	½ cup	13.0
(Greenwood's) red, solids & liq.	½ cup	13.0
Frozen (Green Giant) stuffed	7 oz. serving	16.5
CABERNET SAUVIGNON (Paul,		
Masson)	1 fl. oz.	.2
CAFE COMFORT, 55 proof	1 fl. oz.	8.8
CAKE:		
Regular, non-frozen:		
Plain, home recipe, with butter,		
with boiled white icing	⅑ of 9" square	70.5
Angel food, home recipe	1/12 of 8" cake	24.1
Caramel, home recipe, with		

Food and Description	Measure or Quantity	Carbohydrates (grams)
caramel icing	⅑ of 9″ square	50.2
Carrot (Hostess)	3-oz. piece	28.4
Chocolate, home recipe, with chocolate icing, 2-layer	¹⁄₁₂ of 9″ cake	55.2
Crumb (Hostess)	1¼-oz. cake	21.7
Fruit:		
Home recipe, dark	¹⁄₃₀ of 8″ loaf	9.0
Home recipe, light, made with butter	¹⁄₃₀ of 8″ loaf	8.6
(Holland Honey Cake) unsalted	¹⁄₁₄ of cake	19.0
Pound, home recipe, traditional, made with butter	3½″ × 3½″ slice	16.4
Raisin date loaf (Holland Honey Cake) low sodium	¹⁄₁₄ of 13-oz. cake	19.0
Sponge, home recipe	¹⁄₁₂ of 10″ cake	35.7
White, home recipe, made with butter, without icing, 2-layer	⅑ of 9″ wide, 3″ high cake	50.8
Yellow, home recipe, made with butter, without icing, 2-layer	¹⁄₁₉ of cake	56.3
Frozen:		
Apple walnut:		
(Pepperidge Farm) with cream cheese icing)	⅛ of 11¾-oz. cake	18.0
(Sara Lee	⅛ of 12½-oz. cake	21.6
Banana (Sara Lee)	⅛ of 13 ¾-oz. cake	26.9
Banana nut (Sara Lee) layer	⅛ of 20-oz. cake	26.5
Black forest (Sara Lee)	⅛ of 21-oz. cake	27.9
Boston cream (Pepperidge Farm) Supreme	¼ of 11¾-oz. cake	39.0
Carrot (Sara Lee)	⅛ of 12¼-oz. cake	18.9
Cheesecake:		
(Morton) *Great Little Desserts:*		
Cream	6½-oz. cake	46.2
Strawberry	6½-oz. cake	57.2
(Rich's) Viennese	¹⁄₁₄ of 42-oz. cake	24.1
(Sara Lee):		
Blueberry, *For 2*	½ of 11.3-oz. cake	66.6
Cream cheese	⅓ of 10-oz. cake	29.9
Cream cheese, blueberry	⅙ of 19-oz. cake	35.3
Cream cheese, cherry*	⅙ of 19-oz. cake	35.2
Cream cheese, strawberry	⅙ of 19-oz. cake	33.6
Chocolate:		
(Pepperidge Farm):		
Layer, Fudge	¹⁄₁₀ of 17-oz. cake	23.0

Food and Description	Measure or Quantity	Carbohydrates (grams)
Rich 'N Moist, with chocolate icing	⅛ of 14¼-oz. cake	23.0
(Sara Lee):		
Regular	⅛ of 13¼-oz. cake	28.1
Bavarian	⅛ of 22½-oz. cake	22.6
German	⅛ of 12¼-oz. cake	19.3
Layer, 'n cream	⅛ of 18-oz. cake	23.8
Coffee (Sara Lee):		
Almond ring	⅛ of 9½-oz. cake	16.8
Apple	⅛ of 15-oz. cake	24.1
Apple, *For 2*	½ of 9-oz. cake	58.1
Blueberry ring	⅛ of 9¾-oz. cake	17.6
Maple crunch ring	⅛ of 9¾-oz. cake	17.3
Pecan	¼ of 6½-oz. cake	22.1
Pecan	⅛ of 11¼-oz. cake	19.1
Streusel, butter	⅛ of 11½-oz. cake	20.3
Streusel, cinnamon	⅛ of 10.9-oz. cake	19.0
Crumb (See ROLL OR BUN, Crumb)		
Devil's Food (Pepperidge Farm) layer	⅒ of 17-oz. cake	24.0
Golden (Pepperidge Farm) layer	⅒ of 17-oz. cake	24.0
Orange (Sara Lee)	⅛ of 13¾-oz. cake	25.3
Pineapple cream (Pepperidge Farm) Supreme	1/12 of 24-oz. cake	27.0
Pound (Sara Lee):		
Regular	⅒ of 10¾-oz. cake	14.2
Banana nut	⅒ of 11-oz. cake	15.1
Chocolate	⅒ of 10¾-oz. cake	14.4
Family size	1/15 of 16½-oz. cake	14.8
Homestyle	⅒ of 9½-oz. cake	13.1
Raisin	⅒ of 12.9-oz. cake	19.6
Strawberry cream (Pepperidge Farm) Supreme	1/12 of 24-oz. cake	27.0
Strawberries 'n cream, layer (Sara Lee)	⅛ of 20½-oz. cake	25.9
Torte (Sara Lee):		
Apples 'n cream	⅛ of 21-oz. cake	26.2
Fudge & nut	⅛ of 15¾-oz. cake	21.0
Vanilla (Pepperidge Farm) layer	⅒ of 17-oz. cake	25.0
Walnut, layer (Sara Lee)	⅛ of 18-oz. cake	22.8
CAKE OR COOKIE ICING		
(Pillsbury) all flavors	1 T.	12.0
CAKE ICING:		
Butter pecan (Betty Crocker) *Creamy Deluxe*	1/12 of can	27.0

Food and Description	Measure or Quantity	Carbohydrates (grams)
Caramel, home recipe	4-oz.	86.8
Cherry (Betty Crocker) *Creamy Deluxe*	⅟12 of can	28.0
Chocolate:		
(Betty Crocker) *Creamy Deluxe:*		
Regular or sour cream	⅟12 of can	25.0
Chip	⅟12 of can	27.0
Milk	⅟12 of can	26.0
(Duncan Hines)	⅟12 of can	25.0
(Pillsbury) *Frosting Supreme:*		
Fudge or sour cream	⅟12 of can	24.0
Milk	⅟12 of can	25.0
Coconut almond (Pillsbury) *Frosting Supreme*	⅟12 of can	17.0
Cream cheese:		
(Betty Crocker) *Creamy Deluxe*	⅟12 of can	27.0
(Pillsbury) *Frosting Supreme*	⅟12 of can	27.0
Double dutch (Pillsbury) *Frosting Supreme*	⅟12 of can	24.0
Lemon		
(Betty Crocker) *Sunkist, Creamy Deluxe*	⅟12 of can	28.0
(Pillsbury (*Frosting Supreme*	⅟12 of can	27.0
Orange (Betty Crocker) *Creamy Deluxe*	⅟12 of can	28.0
Strawberry (Pillsbury) *Frosting Supreme*	⅟12 of can	27.0
Vanilla:		
(Betty Crocker) *Creamy Deluxe*	⅟12 of can	28.0
(Duncan Hines)	⅟12 of can	25.5
(Pillsbury) *Frosting Supreme*	⅟12 of can	27.0
White:		
Home recipe, boiled	4 oz.	91.1
Home recipe, uncooked	4 oz.	92.5
(Betty Crocker) *Creamy Deluxe*	⅟12 of can	27.0
*CAKE ICING MIX:		
Regular:		
Banana (Betty Crocker) *Chiquita*, creamy	⅟12 of pkg.	30.0
Butter Brickle (Betty Crocker) creamy	⅟12 of pgk.	30.0
Butter pecan (Betty Crocker) creamy	⅟12 of pkg.	30.0
Caramel (Pillsbury) *Rich'n Easy*	⅟12 of pkg.	24.0
Cherry (Betty Crocker) creamy	⅟12 of pkg.	30.0

Food and Description	Measure or Quantity	Carbohydrates (grams)
Chocolate:		
Home recipe, fudge	½ cup	103.8
(Betty Crocker) creamy:		
Fluffy, almond fudge	1/12 of pkg.	27.0
Fudge, regular, dark or milk	1/12 of pkg.	30.0
(Pillsbury) *Rich 'N Easy:*		
Fudge	1/12 of pkg.	27.0
Milk	1/12 of pkg.	26.0
Coconut almond (Pillsbury)	1/12 of pkg.	16.0
Coconut pecan:		
(Betty Crocker) creamy	1/12 of pkg.	18.0
(Pillsbury)	1/12 of pkg.	20.0
Cream cheese & nut		
(Betty Crocker) creamy	1/12 of pkg.	24.0
Double dutch (Pillsbury)		
Rich 'N Easy	1/12 of pkg.	26.0
Lemon:		
(Betty Crocker) *Sunkist,* creamy	1/12 of pkg.	30.0
(Pillsbury) *Rich 'N Easy*	1/12 of pkg.	25.0
Strawberry (Pillsbury)		
Rich 'N Easy	1/12 of pkg.	25.0
Vanilla (Pillsbury) *Rich 'N Easy*	1/12 of pkg.	25.0
White:		
(Betty Crocker) fluffy	1/12 of pkg.	16.0
(Pillsbury) fluffy	1/12 of pkg.	15.0
Dietetic (Betty Crocker) *Lite,* chocolate, lemon or vanilla	1/12 of pkg.	19.0
CAKE MIX:		
Regular:		
Angel Food:		
(Betty Crocker):		
Chocolate or One-Step	1/12 pkg.	32.0
Traditional	1/12 pkg.	30.0
(Duncan Hines)	1/12 pkg.	28.9
*(Pillsbury) raspberry or white	1/12 of cake	33.0
Applesauce raisin (Betty Crocker) *Snackin' Cake*	1/9 pkg.	33.0
*Applesauce spice (Pillsbury) *Pillsbury Plus*	1/12 of cake	36.0
Banana:		
*(Betty Crocker) *Super Moist*	1/12 of cake	36.0
*(Pillsbury) *Pillsbury Plus*	1/12 of cake	36.0
Banana walnut (Betty Crocker) *Snackin' Cake*	1/9 pkg.	31.0
*Butter (Pillsbury):		
Pillsbury Plus	1/12 of cake	36.0

Food and Description	Measure or Quantity	Carbohydrates (grams)
Streusel Swirl, rich	1/16 of cake	38.0
*Butter Brickle (Betty Crocker)		
Super Moist	1/12 of cake	37.0
*Butter pecan (Betty Crocker)		
Super Moist	1/12 of cake	35.0
*Butter yellow (Betty Crocker)		
Super Moist	1/12 of cake	42.0
*Carrot (Betty Crocker)		
Super Moist	1/12 of cake	34.0
*Carrot 'n spice (Pillsbury)		
Pillsbury Plus	1/12 of cake	36.0
*Cheesecake:		
(Jell-O)	1/8 of 8" cake	33.0
(Royal)	1/8 of cake	31.0
*Cherry chip (Betty Crocker)		
Super Moist	1/12 of cake	36.0
Chocolate:		
(Betty Crocker):		
*Pudding	1/6 of cake	45.0
Snackin' Cake:		
Almond	1/9 pkg.	31.0
Fudge chip	1/9 pkg.	32.0
Stir 'N Frost:		
with chocolate frosting	1/6 pkg.	40.0
Fudge, with vanilla frosting	1/6 pkg.	41.0
Super Moist:		
*Fudge	1/12 of cake	35.0
*German	1/12 of cake	36.0
*Sour cream	1/12 of cake	36.0
*(Pillsbury):		
Bundt:		
Fudge nut crown	1/16 of cake	31.0
Fudge, tunnel of	1/16 of cake	37.0
Macaroon	1/16 of cake	37.0
Pillsbury Plus:		
Fudge, dark	1/12 of cake	35.0
Fudge, marble	1/12 of cake	36.0
German	1/12 of cake	36.0
Mint	1/12 of cake	35.0
Streusel Swirl, German	1/16 of cake	36.0
Cinnamon (Betty Crocker)		
Stir 'N Streusel	1/6 of pkg.	42.0
Coconut pecan (Betty Crocker)		
Snackin' Cake	1/9 of pkg.	30.0
Coffee cake:		
*(Aunt Jemima)	1/8 of cake	29.0

Food and Description	Measure or Quantity	Carbohydrates (grams)
*(Pillsbury):		
Apple cinnamon	⅛ of cake	40.0
Cinnamon streusel	⅛ of cake	41.0
Date nut (Betty Crocker)		
Snackin' Cake	⅑ of pkg.	32.0
Devil's food:		
*(Betty Crocker) *Super Moist*	1/12 of cake	34.0
(Duncan Hines) deluxe	1/12 of pkg.	35.6
*(Pillsbury), *Pillsbury Plus*	1/12 of cake	35.0
Fudge (See Chocolate)		
Golden chocolate chip		
(Betty Crocker) *Snackin' Cake*	⅑ of pkg.	34.0
Lemon:		
(Betty Crocker):		
*Chiffon	1/12 of cake	35.0
Stir 'N Frost, with		
lemon frosting	1/12 of pkg.	39.0
Super Moist	1/12 of cake	36.0
*(Pillsbury):		
Bundt, tunnel of	1/16 of cake	45.0
Streusel Swirl	1/16 of cake	39.0
*Lemon blueberry (Pillsbury)		
Bundt	1/16 of cake	28.0
Marble:		
*(Betty Crocker) *Super Moist*	1/12 of cake	36.0
*(Pillsbury):		
Bundt, supreme, ring	1/16 of cake	38.0
Streusel Swirl, fudge	1/16 of cake	38.0
*Orange (Betty Crocker)		
Super Moist	1/12 of cake	36.0
Pound:		
*(Betty Crocker) golden	1/12 of cake	27.0
*(Dromedary)	¾" slice	29.0
*(Pillsbury) *Bundt*	1/16 of cake	33.0
Spice (Betty Crocker):		
Snackin' Cake, raisin	⅑ of pkg.	32.0
Super Moist	1/12 of cake	36.0
Strawberry:		
*(Betty Crocker) *Supermoist*	1/12 of cake	36.0
*(Pillsbury) *Pillsbury Plus*	1/12 of cake	37.0
*Upside down (Betty Crocker)		
pineapple	⅑ of cake	43.0
White:		
(*Betty Crocker)		
Stir 'N Frost, with chocolate		
frosting	⅙ of cake	38.0

Food and Description	*Measure or Quantity*	*Carbohydrates (grams)*
Super Moist	1/12 of cake	35.0
(Duncan Hines) deluxe	1/12 of pkg.	36.1
*(Pillsbury) *Pillsbury Plus*	1/12 of cake	35.0
Yellow:		
*(Betty Crocker) *Supermoist*	1/12 of cake	36.0
(Duncan Hines) deluxe	1/12 of pkg.	37.0
*(Pillsbury) *Pillsbury Plus*	1/12 of cake	36.0
*Dietetic		
Chocolate	1/10 of cake	20.7
Lemon	1/10 of cake	19.1
White	1/10 of cake	17.9
CAMPARI	1 fl. oz.	7.1
CANDY, REGULAR:		
Almond, chocolate covered (Hershey's) *Golden Almond*	1 oz.	12.4
Almond Cluster (Heath)	1 oz.	17.0
Almond, Jordan (Banner	1¼-oz. box	27.9
Apricot Delight (Sahadi)	1 oz.	25.0
Baby Ruth	1.8-oz. piece	31.0
Bridge mix (Nabisco)	1 piece	1.4
Bun Bars (Wayne)	1 oz.	17.0
Butter Brickle Bar (Heath)	1 oz.	17.0
Butterfinger,	1.6-oz. bar	28.0
Butterscotch Skimmers (Nabisco)	1 piece	5.7
Caramel:		
Caramel Flipper (Wayne)	1 oz.	19.0
Caramel Nip (Pearson)	1 piece	5.6
Caramel Pattie (Heath)	1-oz. serving	17.0
Cereal Raisin Bar (Heath)	2-oz. serving	37.0
Charleston Chew	1½-oz. bar	32.6
Cherry, chocolate-covered (Nabisco; *Welch's*)	1 piece	13.0
Chocolate bar:		
Choco-Lite (Nestlé)	.27-oz. bar	4.9
Choco-Lite (Nestlé)	1-oz. serving	18.0
Crunch (Nestlé)	1 1/16-oz. bar	19.1
Krunch (Heath)	1½-oz. serving	28.0
Milk:		
(Heath) crunch with toffee	2¼-oz. serving	42.0
(Heath) solid	2¼-oz. serving	41.0
(Hershey's)	1.2-oz. bar	19.4
(Hershey's)	4-oz. bar	64.7
(Nestlé)	.35-oz. bar	6.0
(Nestlé)	1 1/16-oz. bar	18.1
Special Dark (Hershey's)	1.05-oz. bar	18.4

Food and Description	Measure or Quantity	Carbohydrates (grams)
Special Dark (Hershey's)	4-oz. bar	70.2
Chocolate bar with almonds:		
(Heath)	2½-oz. serving	39.0
(Hershey's) milk	.35-oz. bar	5.4
(Hershey's) milk	1.15-oz. bar	17.6
(Hershey's) milk	4-oz. bar	61.4
(Nestlé)	1-oz. serving	17.0
Chocolate Parfait (Pearson)	1 piece	5.2
Chuckles	1 oz.	23.0
Clark Bar	1.4-oz. bar	28.4
Coffee Nip (Pearson)	1 piece	5.6
Coffioca (Pearson)	1 piece	5.2
Crispy Bar (Clark)	1¼-oz. bar	24.2
Crows (Mason)	1 piece	2.7
Dots (Mason)	1 piece	2.7
Dutch Treat Bar (Clark)	1¹⁄₁₆-oz. bar	20.3
Fudge (Nabisco) bar, *Home Style*	1 bar	13.9
Good & Plenty	1 oz.	24.8
Halvah (Sahadi) original & marble	1 oz.	13.0
Hollywood	1½-oz. bar	28.9
Jelly bean (Curtiss)	1 piece	3.0
Jujubes, Chuckles	1 piece	3.3
Ju Jus:		
Assorted	1 piece	2.0
Coins or raspberries	1 piece	4.0
Kisses (Hershey's)	1 piece	2.8
Kit Kat	.6-oz. bar	9.4
Krackel Bar	.35-oz. bar	5.9
Krackel Bar	1.2-oz. bar	20.3
Licorice:		
Licorice Nips (Pearson)	1 piece	5.6
(Switzer) bars, bites or stix:		
Black	1 oz.	22.1
Cherry or strawberry	1 oz.	23.2
Chocolate	1 oz.	22.7
Lollipops (Life Savers)	.9-oz. pop	24.0
Mallo Cup (Boyer)	⁹⁄₁₆-oz. piece	11.2
Malted milk balls (Brach's)	1 piece	.9
Mars Bar (M&M/Mars)	1½-oz. serving	26.0
Marshmallow (Campfire)	1 oz.	24.9
Mary Jane (Miller):		
Small size	¼ oz.	3.5
Large size	1½ oz.	20.3
Milk Duds (Clark)	¾-oz. box	17.8
Milk Duds (Clark)	1¼-oz. box.	29.6
Milky Way (M&M/Mars)	.8-oz. bar	16.5

26

Food and Description	Measure or Quantity	Carbohydrates (grams)
Milky Way (M&M/Mars)	1.9-oz. serving	39.2
Mint or peppermint:		
Jamaica or *Liberty Mints*		
(Nabisco)	1 piece	5.8
Meltaway (Heath)	1 oz.	16.0
Mint Parfait (Pearson)	1 piece	5.2
Junior mint pattie (Nabisco)	1 piece	2.0
Peppermint pattie (Nabisco)	1 piece	12.5
M & M's:		
Peanut	1½ oz.	25.0
Plain	1½ oz.	29.0
Mr. Goodbar (Hershey's)	.35-oz. bar	4.9
Mr. Goodbar (Hershey's)	1½-oz. bar	20.8
$100,000 Bar (Nestlé)	1¼-oz. bar	23.8
Orange slices (Curtiss)	1 piece	7.2
Peanut, chocolate-covered:		
(Curtiss)	1 piece	1.0
(Nabisco)	1 piece	1.6
Peanut brittle (Planters):		
Jumbo Peanut Block Bar	1 oz.	23.0
Jumbo Peanut Block Bar	1 piece (4 grams)	12.0
Peanut butter cup:		
(Boyer)	1.5-oz. pkg.	17.4
(Reese's)	.6-oz. cup	8.7
Raisin, chocolate-covered, (Nabisco)	1 piece	.6
Reggie Bar	2-oz. bar	29.0
Rolo (Hershey's)	1 piece	4.1
Royals, mint chocolate (M&M/Mars)	1½-oz. serving	29.2
Sesame crunch (Sahadi)	¾-oz. bar	7.0
Snickers	1.8-oz. bar	30.7
Starburst (M&M/Mars)	1.9-oz. serving	24.2
Sugar Babies (Nabisco)	1 piece	1.3
Sugar Daddy (Nabisco):		
Caramel sucker	1 piece	26.4
Nugget	1 piece	6.0
Sugar Mama (Nabisco)	1 piece	18.6
Summit, cookie bar (M&M/Mars)	1-oz. serving	15.7
Taffy, Turkish (Bonomo)	1-oz. bar	24.4
3 Muskateers	.8-oz. bar	17.3
3 Muskateers	2-oz. serving	44.6
Toffee Brickle (Heath)	1 oz.	17.0
Tootsie Roll:		
Chocolate	.23-oz. midgee	5.3
Chocolate	¹⁄₁₆-oz. bar	14.3
Chocolate	¾-oz. bar	17.2
Chocolate	1-oz. bar	22.9

Food and Description	Measure or Quantity	Carbohydrates (grams)
Chocolate	1¾-oz. bar	40.0
Flavored	.6-oz. square	3.8
Pop, all flavors	.49-oz. pop	12.5
Pop drop, all flavors	4.7-gram piece	4.2
Twix, cookie bar (M&M/Mars)	1¾-oz. serving	32.6
Twix, peanut butter cookie bar (M&M/Mars)	1¾-oz. serving	27.9
Twizzlers:		
Cherry, chocolate or strawberry	1 oz.	21.0
Licorice	1 oz.	20.0
Whatchamacallit (Hershey's)	1.15-oz. bar	18.7
World Series Bar	1 oz.	21.3
Zagnut Bar (Clark)	.7-oz. bar	14.6
CANDY, DIETETIC:		
Carob bar, *Joan's Natural:*		
Coconut	1 section of 3-oz. bar	2.4
Coconut	3-oz. bar	28.4
Fruit & nut	1 section of 3-oz. bar	2.6
Fruit & nut	3-oz. bar	31.2
Honey bran	1 section of 3-oz. bar	2.8
Honey bran	3-oz. bar	34.0
Peanut	1 section of 3-oz. bar	2.3
Peanut	3-oz. bar	27.4
Chocolate or chocolate flavored bar, (Estee):		
Bittersweet	1 section of 2½-oz. bar	2.7
Bittersweet	2½-oz. bar	32.0
Coconut	1 section of 2½-oz. bar	7.4
Coconut	2½-oz. bar	88.3
Crunch	1 section of 2-oz. bar	2.7
Crunch	2-oz. bar	32.2
Fruit & nut	1 section of 2½-oz. bar	2.6
Fruit & nut	2½-oz. bar	31.3
Milk	1 section of 2½-oz. bar	2.6
Milk	2½-oz. bar	31.0
Toasted bran	1 section of 2½-oz. bar	2.7
Toasted bran	2½-oz. bar	32.6
Chocolate bar with almonds (Estee) milk	1 section of 2½-oz. bar	2.4

Food and Description	Measure or Quantity	Carbohydrates (grams)
Chocolate bar with almonds (Estee) milk	2½-oz. bar	29.2
Estee-ets, with peanuts (Estee)	1 piece	.9
Gum drops (Estee) any flavor	1 piece	.7
Hard candy:		
(Estee) assorted fruit or peppermint	1 piece	2.7
(Estee) Tropi-mix	1 piece	2.7
Mint:		
(Estee) *Esteemints*, all flavors	1 piece	1.1
(Sunkist):		
Mini mint	1 piece	.2
Roll mint	1 piece	.9
Peanut butter cup (Estee)	1 cup	3.3
Raisins, chocolate-covered (Estee)	1 piece	.6
CANNELLONI FLORENTINE, frozen		
(Weight Watchers) one-compartment	13-oz. meal	52.0
CANTALOUPE, cubed	½ cup	6.1
CAP'N CRUNCH cereal (Quaker):		
Regular or crunchberry	¾ cup	22.9
Peanut butter	¾ cup	20.9
CARAWAY SEED (French's)	1 tsp.	.8
CARNATION INSTANT BREAKFAST:		
Bar:		
Chocolate chip	1 bar	21.0
Peanut butter crunch	1 bar	20.0
Dry, coffee, strawberry or vanilla	1 packet	24.0
CARROT:		
Raw	5½″ × 1″ carrot	2.8
Boiled, slices, without salt	½ cup	5.8
Canned, regular:		
(Del Monte) drained	½ cup	6.0
(Libby's) solids & liq.	½ cup	4.1
(Stokely-Van Camp) solids & liq.	½ cup	5.0
Canned, dietetic:		
(Featherweight) solids & liq.	½ cup	6.0
(S&W) *Nutradiet*, sliced, solids & liq.	½ cup	7.0
Frozen:		
(Birds Eye) with brown sugar glaze	⅓ pkg.	15.3
(Green Giant) cuts in butter sauce	⅓ pkg.	16.0
(McKenzie)	⅓ pkg.	9.0
(Seabrook Farms)	⅓ pkg.	8.1
CASABA MELON	1-lb. melon	14.7

Food and Description	Measure or Quantity	Carbohydrates (grams)
CASHEW NUT:		
(Fisher):		
Dry roasted	1 oz.	8.2
Oil roasted	1 oz.	8.3
(Planters):		
Dry roasted, salted	1 oz.	9.0
Oil roasted, salted	1 oz.	8.0
CATSUP:		
Regular:		
(Del Monte)	1 T.	3.9
(Smucker's)	1 T.	4.5
(Dietetic:		
(Featherweight)	1 T.	1.0
(Tillie Lewis) *Tasti Diet*	1 T.	2.0
CAULIFLOWER:		
Raw or boiled buds	½ cup	2.6
Frozen:		
(Birds Eye) florets, deluxe	⅓ pkg.	4.6
(Green Giant) in cheese sauce,	⅓ pkg.	8.1
(Mrs. Paul's) light batter & cheese	⅓ pkg.	15.3
(Seabrook Farms)	⅓ pkg.	4.5
(Stouffer's) au gratin	5-oz. serving	10.9
CAVIAR:		
Pressed	1 oz.	1.4
Whole eggs	1 T.	.5
CELERY:		
1 large outer stalk	8″ × 1½″ at root end	1.6
Diced or cut	½ cup	2.1
Salt (French's)	1 piece	Tr.
CERTS	1 piece	1.5
CHABLIS WINE:		
(Great Western)	3 fl. oz.	2.0
(Paul Masson), regular or light	3 fl. oz.	2.7
CHAMPAGNE:		
(Great Western):		
Regular	3 fl. oz.	2.4
Brut	3 fl. oz.	3.4
Extra dry	3 fl. oz.	4.3
Pink	3 fl. oz.	4.9
(Taylor) dry	3 fl. oz.	3.3
CHARLOTTE RUSSE,		
homemade recipe	4 oz.	38.0
CHEERIOS, cereal (General Mills):		
Regular	1¼ cup	20.0
Honey nut	¾ cup	23.0

Food and Description	Measure or Quantity	Carbohydrates (grams)
CHEESE:		
American or cheddar:		
Cube, natural	1″ cube	.4
Laughing Cow	1 oz.	Tr.
(Sargento):		
Midget, regular or sharp	1 oz.	1.0
Shredded, non-dairy	1 oz.	1.0
Wispride, sharp	1 oz.	1.0
Blue:		
(Frigo)	1 oz.	1.0
Laughing Cow:		
Cube	⅙ oz.	.1
Wedge	¾ oz.	.5
(Sargento): cold pack or crumbled	1 oz.	1.0
Brick (Sargento)	1 oz.	1.0
Brie (Sargento) *Danish Danko*	1 oz.	.1
Burgercheese (Sargento)		
Danish Danko	1 oz.	1.0
Camembert (Sargento)		
Danish Danko	1 oz.	.1
Colby:		
(Featherweight) low sodium	1 oz.	0.
(Pauly) low sodium	1 oz.	
(Sargento) shredded or sliced	1 oz.	1.0
Cottage:		
Unflavored:		
(Bison):		
Regular	1 oz.	1.0
Dietetic	1 oz.	1.0
(Dairylea)	1 oz.	1.0
(Friendship)	1 oz.	1.0
Flavored (Friendship):		
With Dutch apple	1 oz.	2.5
With garden salad	1 oz.	1.0
With pineapple	1 oz.	3.8
Cream, plain, unwhipped:		
(Frigo)	1 oz.	1.0
Philadelphia (Kraft)	1 oz.	.9
Edam:		
(House of Gold)	1 oz.	1.0
Laughing Cow	1 oz.	Tr.
(Sargento)	1 oz.	1.0
Farmers:		
Dutch Garden Brand	1 oz.	1.0
(Friendship) regular or no salt		
added	1 oz.	1.0

Food and Description	Measure or Quantity	Carbohydrates (grams)
(Sargento)	1 oz.	1.0
Wispride	1 oz.	1.0
Feta (Sargento) Danish, cups	1 oz.	1.0
Gjetost (Sargento) Norwegian	1 oz.	13.0
Gouda:		
(Frigo)	1 oz.	1.0
Laughing Cow, natural	1 oz.	Tr.
(Sargento) baby, caraway or smoked	1 oz.	1.0
Wispride	1 oz.	<1.0
Gruyere, *Swiss Knight*	1 oz.	<1.0
Havarti (Sargento):		
Creamy	1 oz.	.2
Creamy, 60% mild	1 oz.	.2
Hot pepper (Sargento)	1 oz.	1.0
Jarlsberg (Sargento) Norwegian	1 oz.	1.0
Kettle Moraine (Sargento)	1 oz.	1.0
Limburger (Sargento) natural	1 oz.	14.0
Monterey Jack:		
(Frigo)	1 oz.	1.0
(Sargento) Midget, Longhorn, shredded or sliced	1 oz.	1.0
Mozzarella:		
(Fisher) part skim milk	1 oz.	1.0
(Sargento):		
Bar, rounds, shredded, shredded with spices, sliced for pizza or square	1 oz.	1.0
Whole milk	1 oz.	1.0
Muenster:		
(Sargento) red rind	1 oz.	1.0
(*Wispride*	1 oz.	<1.0
Nibblin Curds (Sargento)	1 oz.	1.0
Parmesan:		
(Frigo):		
Grated	1 T.	Tr.
Whole	1 oz.	1.0
(Sargento):		
Grated	1 T.	2.3
Wedge	1 oz.	1.0
Pizza (Sargento) shredded or sliced	1 oz.	1.0
Pot (Sargento) regular, French onion or garlic	1 oz.	1.0
Provolone:		
(Frigo)	1 oz.	1.0

Food and Description	Measure or Quantity	Carbohydrates (grams)
Laughing Cow:		
Cube	⅙ oz.	.1
Wedge	¾ oz.	.5
(Sargento) sliced	1 oz.	1.0
Ricotta:		
(Frigo) part skim milk	1 oz.	.9
(Sargento):		
Part skim milk	1 oz.	1.0
Whole milk	1 oz.	1.0
Romano (Sargento) wedge	1 oz.	1.0
Roquefort, natural	1 oz.	.6
Samsoe (Sargento) Danish	1 oz.	.2
Scamorze (Frigo)	1 oz.	.3
Stirred Curd (Frigo)	1 oz.	1.0
String (Sargento)	1 oz.	1.0
Swiss:		
(Fisher) natural	1 oz.	0.
(Frigo) domestic	1 oz.	0.
(Sargento) domestic, or Finland, sliced	1 oz.	1.0
Taco (Sargento) shredded	1 oz.	1.0
Washed curd (Frigo)	1 oz.	1.0
CHEESE FONDUE, *Swiss Knight*	1-oz. serving	1.0
CHEESE FOOD:		
American or cheddar:		
(Weight Watchers) colored or white	1-oz. slice	1.0
Wispride:		
Regular	1 oz.	2.0
& blue cheese	1 oz.	2.0
Hickory smoked	1 oz.	3.0
& port wine	1 oz.	<1.0
Cheez 'N Crackers (Kraft)	1 piece	9.3
Cheez-ola (Fisher)	1 oz.	.5
Cracker Snack (Sargento)	1 oz.	2.0
Loaf, *Count Down* (Pauly)	1 oz.	3.0
Mun-chee (Pauly)	1 oz.	2.0
Pimiento (Pauly)	.8-oz. slice	.8
Swiss (Pauly)	.8-oz. slice	1.6
CHEESE PUFFS, frozen (Durkee)	1 piece	3.0
CHEESE SPREAD:		
American or cheddar:		
(Fisher)	1 oz.	2.0
(Nabisco) *Snack Mate*	1 tsp.	.4
Cheese 'n Bacon (Nabisco) *Snack Mate*	1 tsp.	.4

Food and Description	Measure or Quantity	Carbohydrates (grams)
Cheez Whiz (Kraft)	1 oz.	1.8
Count Down (Fisher)	1 oz.	3.0
Imitation (Fisher) *Chef's Delight*	1 oz.	3.0
Pimiento:		
(Nabisco) *Snack Mate*	1 tsp.	.3
(Price's)	1 oz.	2.0
Sharp (Pauly)	.8 oz.	.9
Swiss, process (Pauly)	.8 oz.	1.2
Velveeta (Kraft)	1 oz.	2.5
CHEESE STRAW, frozen (Durkee)	1 piece	1.0
CHERRY, sweet:		
Fresh, with stems	½ cup	10.2
Canned, regular (Stokely-Van Camp) pitted, solids & liq.	½ cup	11.0
Canned, dietetic, solids & liq.:		
(Diet Delight) with pits, water pack	½ cup	17.0
(Featherweight) dark, water pack	½ cup	13.0
(Featherweight) light, water pack	½ cup	11.0
CHERRY, CANDIED	1 oz.	24.6
CHERRY DRINK:		
Canned:		
(Hi-C)	6 fl. oz.	23.0
(Lincoln) cherry berry	6 fl. oz.	25.0
*Mix (Hi-C)	6 fl. oz.	18.0
CHERRY HEERING (Hiram Walker)	1 fl. oz.	10.0
CHERRY JELLY:		
Sweetened (Smucker's)	1 T.	13.5
Dietetic:		
(Featherweight)	1 T.	4.0
(Slenderella)	1 T.	6.0
CHERRY LIQUEUR (DeKuyper)	1 fl. oz.	8.5
CHERRY PRESERVE OR JAM:		
Sweetened (Smucker's)	1 T.	6.0
Dietetic:		
(Featherweight) imitation	1 T.	1.0
(S&W) *Nutradiet*, red, tart	1 T.	3.0
CHERRY SPREAD, low sugar (Smucker's)	1 T.	6.0
CHESTNUT, fresh, in shell	¼ lb.	47.7
CHEWING GUM:		
Sweetened:		
Bazooka, bubble	1¢ slice	4.5
Beechies, Chiclets, tiny size	1 piece	1.6

Food and Description	Measure or Quantity	Carbohydrates (grams)
Beech Nut; Beeman's; Big Red; Black Jack; Clove; Doublemint; Freedent; Fruit Punch; Juicy Fruit; Spearmint (Wrigley's); *Teaberry*	1 stick	2.3
Dentyne	1 piece	1.2
Dietetic:		
Bazooka, sugarless	1 piece	Tr.
(Clark; *Care*Free*)	1 piece	1.7
(Estee) bubble or regular	1 piece	1.4
CHEX, cereal (Ralston Purina):		
Rice	1 cup	25.0
Wheat	⅔ cup	23.0
Wheat & raisins	¾ cup	31.0
CHIANTI WINE, (Italian Swiss Colony)	3 fl. oz.	1.5
CHICKEN:		
Broiler, cooked, meat only	3 oz.	0.
Fryer, fried, meat & skin	3 oz.	2.4
Fryer, fried, meat only	3 oz.	1.1
Fryer, fried, a 2½ lb. chicken (weighed with bone before cooking) will give you:		
Back	1 back	2.7
Breast	½ breast	1.2
Leg or drumstick	1 leg	.4
Neck	1 neck	2.0
Rib	1 rib	.8
Thigh	1 thigh	1.3
Wing	1 wing	.8
Fried skin	1 oz.	2.6
Hen & cock:		
Stewed, meat & skin	3 oz.	0.
Stewed, dark meat only	3 oz.	0.
Stewed, light meat only	3 oz.	0.
Stewed, diced	½ cup	0.
Roaster, roasted, dark or light meat without skin	3 oz.	0.
CHICKEN A LA KING:		
Home recipe	1 cup	12.3
Canned (Swanson)	½ of 10½-oz. can	9.0
Frozen:		
(Banquet) *Cookin' Bag*	5-oz. pkg.	10.4
(Green Giant) *Toast Topper*	5-oz. pkg.	
(Stouffer's) with rice	½ of 9½-oz. pkg.	18.9
(Weight Watchers)	10-oz. bag	17.0

Food and Description	Measure or Quantity	Carbohydrates (grams)
CHICKEN BOUILLON:		
(Herb-Ox):		
Cube	1 cube	.6
Packet	1 packet	1.9
(Maggi)	1 cube	1.0
Low sodium (Featherweight)	1 tsp.	2.0
CHICKEN BONED, CANNED		
(Swanson)	Any quantity	0.
CHICKEN, CREAMED, frozen		
(Stouffer's)	6½ oz.	5.9
CHICKEN DINNER OR ENTREE:		
Canned (Swanson) & dumplings	7½ oz.	19.0
Frozen:		
(Banquet):		
Regular:		
& dumplings	12-oz. dinner	36.4
Fried	11-oz. dinner	48.4
Buffet Supper	2-lb. pkg.	128.2
Man-Pleaser:		
& dressing	19-oz. dinner	68.4
& dumplings	19-oz. dinner	86.1
(Green Giant):		
& broccoli with rice in cheese sauce	10-oz. entree	27.8
& pea pods, in sauce with rice & vegetables	10-oz. entree	35.2
(Morton):		
Boneless	10-oz. dinner	22.8
Country Table	15-oz. dinner	94.8
Country Table, fried	12-oz. entree	27.3
& dumplings	11-oz. dinner	31.2
(Mrs. Paul's) pattie, breaded & fried with french fries	8½-oz. pkg.	51.3
(Stouffer's):		
Cacciatore, with spaghetti	11¼-oz. meal	28.8
Divan	8½-oz. serving	14.0
(Swanson):		
Regular, in white wine sauce	8¼-oz. entree	8.0
Hungry Man:		
Boneless	19-oz. dinner	65.0
Fried, white portion	15¼-oz. dinner	90.0
TV Brand, fried:		
Barbecue	11¼-oz. dinner	50.0
Nibbles	6-oz. entree	30.0
White portion	11½-oz. dinner	48.0
3-course, fried	15-oz. dinner	53.0

Food and Description	Measure or Quantity	Carbohydrates (grams)
(Weight Watchers):		
New Orleans style	11-oz. bag	19.1
Oriental style	12-oz. bag	18.0
Parmigiana, 2-compartment	7¾-oz. pkg.	11.0
Sliced, with gravy & stuffing, 3-compartment	14¾-oz. pkg.	42.1
Sweet 'n Sour	9½-oz. bag	27.0
CHICKEN, FRIED, frozen:		
(Banquet)	2-lb. bag	117.3
(Morton)	2-lb. bag	163.5
(Swanson):		
Assorted pieces	3.2-oz. serving	11.0
Breast	3.2-oz. serving	15.0
Nibbles (wing)	3.2-oz. serving	16.0
Take-out style	4-oz. serving	10.0
CHICKEN LIVER, & ONION, frozen		
(Weight Watchers) 2-compartment	9¼-oz. meal	10.0
CHICKEN & NOODLES:		
Frozen:		
(Banquet) *Buffet Supper*	2-lb. pkg.	79.1
(Green Giant) with vegetables	9-oz. pkg.	34.3
CHICKEN, PACKAGED,		
(Louis Rich) breast, oven roasted	1-oz. slice	<1.0
CHICKEN PIE, frozen:		
(Banquet) regular	8-oz. pie	39.0
(Morton)	8-oz. pie	29.5
(Stouffer's)	10-oz. pie	39.8
(Swanson):		
Regular	8-oz. pie	40.0
Hungry Man	1-lb. pie	65.0
(Van de Kamp's)	7½-oz. pie	47.0
CHICKEN PUFF (Durkee)	½-oz. piece	3.0
CHICKEN SALAD (Carnation)	1½-oz. serving	3.8
CHICKEN SOUP (*See* SOUP, Chicken)		
CHICKEN SPREAD:		
(Swanson)	1-oz. serving	2.0
(Underwood)	1-oz. serving	1.7
CHICKEN STEW, canned:		
Regular:		
(Libby's) with dumpings	8-oz. serving	20.2
(Swanson)	7⅝-oz. serving	16.0
Dietetic (Featherweight)	7¼-oz. can	21.0
CHICKEN STOCK BASE (French's)	1 tsp.	1.0
CHICK-FIL-A:		
Sandwich	5.4-oz. serving	40.2

Food and Description	Measure or Quantity	Carbohydrates (grams)
Soup, hearty:		
Small	8.5 oz.	11.1
Large	14.3 oz.	19.3
CHICK'N QUICK (Tyson):		
Breast fillet	3 oz.	12.0
Breast pattie	3 oz.	11.0
Chick'n Cheddar	3 oz.	12.0
Cordon bleu	5 oz.	16.0
Italian hogie	3 oz.	12.0
Kiev	5 oz.	16.0
CHILI OR CHILI CON CARNE:		
Canned, regular pack:		
Beans only (Van Camp) Mexican style	1 cup	900
With beans:		
(Libby's)	½ of 15-oz. can	25.0
(Nalley's) mild or hot	8-oz. serving	27.3
(Swanson)	7¾-oz. serving	28.0
·Without beans:		
(Libby's)	7½-oz.	11.0
(Nalley's) *Big Chunk*	7½-oz. can	19.2
Canned, dietetic pack (Featherweight) With beans	7½-oz.	25.0
Frozen, with beans (Weight Watchers) one-compartment	10-oz. pkg.	32.9
CHILI SAUCE:		
(Ortega) green	1 oz.	1.1
(Featherweight) dietetic	1 T.	2.0
CHILI SEASONING MIX:		
*(Durkee)	1 cup	31.2
(French's) *Chili-O*	1 pkg.	30.0
CHOCO-DILE (Hostess)	2-oz. piece	34.1
CHOCOLATE, BAKING:		
(Baker's):		
Bitter or unsweetened	1 oz.	8.6
Semi-sweet, chips	¼ cup	31.7
Sweetened, *German's*	1 oz.	17.3
(Hershey's):		
Bitter or unsweetened	1 oz.	6.8
Sweetened:		
Dark, chips, regular or mini	1 oz.	17.8
Milk, chips	1 oz.	18.2
Semi-sweet, chips	1 oz.	17.3
(Nestlé):		
Bitter or unsweetened, *Choco-Bake*	1-oz. packet	12.0

Food and Description	Measure or Quantity	Carbohydrates (grams)
Sweet or semi-sweet, morsels	1 oz.	17.0
CHOCOLATE ICE CREAM		
(*See* Ice Cream)		
CHOCOLATE SYRUP (See SYRUP, Chocolate)		
CHOP SUEY, frozen:		
(Banquet) beef:		
Buffet Supper	2-lb. pkg.	39.1
Cookin' Bag	7-oz. bag	9.5
Dinner	12-oz. dinner	38.8
(Stouffer's) beef, with rice	12-oz. pkg.	47.7
*CHOP SUEY SEASONING MIX		
(Durkee)	1¾ cups	21.0
CHOWDER (See SOUP, Chowder)		
CHOW MEIN:		
Canned:		
(Chun King):		
Chicken	8-oz. serving	6.7
Pork, *Divider-Pak*	12-oz. serving	7.0
(Hormel) pork, *Short Orders*	7½-oz. can	13.0
(La Choy):		
Beef	1 cup	5.7
*Beef, bi-pack	1 cup	10.3
Chicken	½ of 1-lb. can	5.0
*Chicken, bi-pack	1 cup	9 3
Meatless	1 cup	5.9
*Mushroom, bi-pack	1 cup	10.7
Pepper Oriental	1 cup	10.2
*Pepper Oriental, bi-pack	1 cup	11.1
*Pork, bi-pack	1 cup	10.6
Shrimp	1 cup	5.7
*Shrimp, bi-pack	1 cup	9.7
Frozen:		
(Banquet)	12-oz. dinner	38.8
(Green Giant) chicken	9-oz. entree	32.0
(La Choy):		
Beef, 5-compartment	11-oz. dinner	52.8
Chicken	11-oz. dinner	53.8
Pepper oriental	11-oz. dinner	54.6
CINNAMON, GROUND (French's)	1 tsp.	1.4
CITRUS COOLER DRINK, canned		
(Hi-C)	6 fl. oz.	23.0
CLAM:		
Raw, all kinds, meat only	1 cup (8 oz.)	13.4
Raw, soft, meat & liq.	1 lb. (weighed in shell)	53.0

Food and Description	Measure or Quantity	Carbohydrates (grams)
Canned, (Doxsee):		
Chopped & minced, solids & liq.	4 oz.	3.2
Frozen (Mrs. Paul's):		
Deviled	3-oz. piece	14.4
Fried	2½ oz.	24.1
CLAMATO COCKTAIL (Mott's)	6 fl. oz.	19.0
CLAM JUICE (Snow)	½ cup	1.2
CLAM SANDWICH, frozen (Mrs. Paul's)	4½-oz. sandwich	54.3
CLARET WINE:		
(Gold Seal)	3 fl. oz.	.4
(Inglenook) Navelle	3 fl. oz.	.3
(Taylor) 12.5% alcohol	3 fl. oz.	2.4
CLORETS, gum or mint	1 piece	1.3
COCOA:		
Dry, unsweetened:		
(Hershey's)	1 T.	2.0
(Sultana)	1 T.	3.5
Mix, regular:		
(Alba '66) instant, all flavors	1 envelope	11.0
(Carnation) all flavors	1-oz. pkg.	22.0
(Hershey's):		
Hot	1 oz.	21.0
Instant	3 T.	17.0
(Nestlé):		
Hot or with mini marshmallows	1 oz.	23.0
Mix, dietetic:		
*(Featherweight)	6 fl. oz.	8.0
(Ovaltine) hot, reduced calorie	.45-oz. pkg.	8.0
Swiss Miss, instant, lite	3 T.	17.0
COCOA KRISPIES, cereal (Kellogg's)	¾ cup	25.0
COCOA PUFFS, cereal (General Mills)	1 oz. (1 cup)	25.0
COCONUT:		
Fresh, meat only	2″ × 2″ × ½″ piece	4.2
Grated or shredded, loosely packed	½ cup	6.1
Dried:		
(Baker's):		
Angel Flake	⅓ cup	10.6
Cookie	⅓ cup	17.1
Premium shred	⅓ cup	12.4
(Durkee) shredded	¼ cup	2.0
COCO WHEATS, cereal	1 T.	9.1
COD, broiled	3 oz.	0.

Food and Description	Measure or Quantity	Carbohydrates (grams)
COFFEE:		
Regular:		
*Max-Pax; Maxwell House Electra Perk, Yuban; Yuban Electra Matic	6 fl. oz.	0.
*Mellow Roast	6 fl. oz.	1.0
Decaffeinated:		
*Brim, regular	6 fl. oz.	5.0
*Decaf; Nescafé	6 fl. oz.	<10.0
*Sanka, regular or electric perk	6 fl. oz.	1.0
*Freeze-dried, Maxim, Sanka, Taster's Choice	6 fl. oz.	1.0
Instant:		
*Decaf (Nestlé); Nescafé, Sunrise	6 fl. oz.	1.0
*Mellow Roast	6 fl. oz.	2.0
*Mix (General Foods)		
International Coffee:		
Cafe Amaretto	6 fl. oz.	7.0
Cafe Vienna	6 fl. oz.	10.3
Irish Mocha Mint	6 fl. oz.	7.4
COFFEE CAKE (See CAKE, Coffee)		
COFFEE LIQUEUR (DeKuyper)	1½ fl. oz.	18.6
COFFEE SOUTHERN	1 fl. oz.	8.8
COLA SOFT DRINK (See SOFT DRINK, Cola)		
COLD DUCK WINE (Great Western) pink	3 fl. oz.	7.7
COLESLAW, solids & liq., made with mayonnaise-type salad dressing	1 cup	8.5
*COLE SLAW MIX (Libby's) Super Slaw)	½ cup	11.0
COLLARDS:		
Leaves, cooked	½ cup	4.8
Canned (Sunshine) chopped, solids & liq.	½ cup	3.8
Frozen:		
(Birds Eye) chopped	⅓ pkg.	4.4
(McKenzie) chopped	3⅓ oz.	1.0
(Southland) chopped	⅕ of 16-oz. pkg.	5.0
COMPLETE CEREAL (Elam's)	1 oz.	17.5
CONCORD WINE:		
(Gold Seal)	3 fl. oz.	9.8
(Mogen David)	3 fl. oz.	16.0
COOKIE, REGULAR:		
Almond Windmill (Nabisco)	1 piece	7.0

Food and Description	Measure or Quantity	Carbohydrates (grams)
Animal:		
(Dixie Belle)	1 piece	1.5
(Keebler):		
Regular	1 piece	1.9
Iced	1 piece	3.9
(Nabisco) *Barnum's Animals*	1 piece	1.9
Apple (Pepperidge Farm)	1 piece	7.6
Apple Crisp (Nabisco)	1 piece	7.0
Apple Spice (Pepperidge Farm)	1 piece	7.6
Apricot Raspberry (Pepperidge Farm)	1 piece	7.6
Assortment:		
(Nabisco) *Mayfair:*		
Crown creme sandwich	1 piece	8.0
Fancy shortbread biscuit	1 piece	3.3
Filigree creme sandwich	1 piece	8.5
Mayfair creme sandwich	1 piece	9.0
Tea time biscuit	1 piece	3.8
(Pepperidge Farm):		
Butter & Seville	1 piece	7.0
Champagne	1 piece	4.0
Chocolate Laced Pirouette	1 piece	4.3
Marseilles	1 piece	6.0
Bordeaux (Pepperidge Farm)	1 piece	5.3
Brownie:		
(Hostess)	1¼-oz. piece	24.1
(Pepperidge Farm) chocolate nut	.4-oz. piece	6.3
(Sara Lee) frozen	⅛ of 13-oz. pkg.	26.1
Brussels (Pepperidge Farm)	1 piece	6.6
Cappucino (Pepperidge Farm)	1 piece	6.0
Chessmen (Pepperidge Farm)	1 piece	6.0
Chocolate & chocolate-covered:		
(Keebler) fudge covered fudge stripes	1 piece	7.0
(Nabisco):		
Famous wafer	1 piece	4.6
Pinwheel, cake	1 piece	21.0
Snap	1 piece	2.8
Chocolate chip:		
(Keebler) *Rich 'N Chips*	1 piece	10.0
(Nabisco):		
Chips Ahoy!	1 piece	7.0
Chocolate	1 piece	7.3
Cookie Little	1 piece	1.0
(Pepperidge Farm):		
Regular	1 piece	6.7

Food and Description	Measure or Quantity	Carbohydrates (grams)
Large	1 piece	18.0
Coconut:		
(Keebler) chocolate drop	1 piece	9.4
(Nabisco) bar, *Bakers Bonus*	1 piece	5.3
Coconut Granola (Pepperidge Farm)	1 piece	6.7
Creme Stick (Dutch Twin) chocolate coated	1 piece	5.0
Date Nut Granola (Pepperidge Farm)	1 piece	6.7
Double chip fudge (Nabisco)		
Bakers Bonus	1 piece	11.0
Fig bar:		
(Keebler)	1 piece	14.0
(Nabisco):		
Fig Newtons	1 piece	11.0
Fig Wheats	1 piece	11.5
Gingerman (Pepperidge Farm)	1 piece	5.0
Gingersnaps (Nabisco) old fashioned	1 piece	5.5
Granola (Pepperidge Farm)	1 piece	16.0
Ladyfinger	3¼″ × 1⅜″ × 1⅛″	7.1
Lido (Pepperidge Farm)	1 piece	10.5
Macaroon, coconut (Nabisco)	1 piece	11.5
Marshmallow:		
(Nabisco):		
Mallomars	1 piece	8.5
Puffs, cocoa covered	1 piece	14.0
Sandwich	1 piece	5.7
Twirls cakes	1 piece	20.0
Milano (Pepperidge Farm)	1 piece	7.0
Mint Milano (Pepperidge Farm)	1 piece	8.3
Molasses (Nabisco) *Pantry*	1 piece	9.5
Molasses Crisp (Pepperidge Farm)	1 piece	4.0
Nilla wafer (Nabisco)	1 piece	3.0
Oatmeal:		
(Keebler) old fashion	1 piece	12.0
(Nabisco):		
Bakers Bonus	1 piece	12.0
Cookie Little	1 piece	1.0
(Pepperidge Farm):		
Irish	1 piece	6.7
Large	1 piece	7.7
Orange Milano (Pepperidge Farm)	1 piece	8.3
Peanut & peanut butter:		
(Nabisco):		
Biscos	1 piece	5.7
Creme pattie	1 piece	8.8
Fudge	1 piece	6.7

43

Food and Description	Measure or Quantity	Carbohydrates (grams)
(Pepperidge Farm) chip, large	1 piece	16.0
Peanut brittle (Nabisco)	1 piece	6.3
Pecan Sandies (Keebler)	1 piece	9.3
Raisin	1 oz.	22.9
Raisin (Nabisco) fruit biscuit	1 piece	12.0
Raisin Bar (Keebler) iced	1 piece	11.0
Raisin Bran (Pepperidge Farm)	1 piece	6.7
Sandwich:		
(Keebler):		
Chocolate fudge	1 piece	12.0
Elfwich	1 piece	8.1
Pitter Patter	1 piece	11.0
Vanilla creme	1 piece	8.5
(Nabisco):		
Brown edges	1 piece	10.0
Cameo creme	1 piece	10.5
Mystic mint	1 piece	11.0
Oreo	1 piece	7.3
Oreo, double stuf	1 piece	9.0
Shortbread or shortcake:		
(Nabisco):		
Cookie Little	1 piece	1.1
Lorna Doone	1 piece	5.0
Melt-A-Way	1 piece	8.0
Pecan	1 piece	8.5
(Pepperidge Farm)	1 piece	8.5
Social Tea, biscuit (Nabisco)	1 piece	3.5
St. Moritz (Pepperidge Farm)	1 piece	6.6
Sugar (Pepperidge Farm) large	1 piece	17.0
Sugar wafer:		
(Dutch Twin) any flavor	1 piece	4.7
(Keebler) *Krisp Kreem*	1 piece	4.2
(Nabisco) *Biscos*	1 piece	2.6
Tahiti (Pepperidge Farm)	1 piece	8.5
COOKIE, DIETETIC (Estee):		
Chocolate chip	1 piece	4.0
Coconut	1 piece	2.7
Fudge	1 piece	3.3
Lemon, thin	1 piece	3.1
Oatmeal raisin	1 piece	3.3
COOKIE CRISP, cereal, any flavor	1 cup	25.0
*COOKIE DOUGH:		
Refrigerated (Pillsbury):		
Chocolate chip or oatmeal	1 cookie	7.3
Peanut Butter	1 cookie	6.3

Food and Description	Measure or Quantity	Carbohydrates (grams)
Frozen (Rich's):		
Chocolate chip	1 cookie	20.3
Oatmeal	1 cookie	18.3
Sugar	1 cookie	17.4
*COOKIE MIX:		
Regular:		
Brownie:		
(Betty Crocker):		
Fudge, regular size	1/16 of pan	22.0
Walnut, family size	1/24 of pan	19.0
(Duncan Hines)	1/24 of pkg.	19.4
(Pillsbury) fudge, regular size	1½" square	10.0
Chocolate chip:		
(Betty Crocker) *Big Batch*	1 cookie	8.0
(Duncan Hines)	1/36 of pkg.	9.1
(Nestlé)	1 cookie	7.5
(Quaker)	1 cookie	8.5
Macaroon, coconut		
(Betty Crocker)	1/24 of pkg.	10.0
Oatmeal:		
(Betty Crocker) *Big Batch*	1 cookie	8.5
(Duncan Hines) raisin	1/36 of pkg.	9.1
(Quaker)	1 cookie	9.4
Peanut butter (Duncan Hines)	1 cookie	7.5
Sugar:		
(Betty Crocker) *Big Batch*	1 cookie	9.0
(Duncan Hines) golden	1/36 of pkg.	8.4
Dietetic (Dia-Mel)	2" cookie	7.0
COOKING SPRAY, *Mazola No Stick*	2-second spray	0.
CORN:		
Fresh, on the cob, boiled	5" × 1¾" ear	16.2
Canned, regular pack:		
(Del Monte):		
Cream style, golden, wet pack	½ cup	19.1
Whole kernel, drained	½ cup	21.2
Whole kernel, vacuum pack	½ cup	21.6
(Festal):		
Cream style, golden, wet pack	½ cup	19.1
Golden, whole kernel, drained	½ cup	21.2
(Green Giant):		
Cream style	4¼ oz.	21.3
Whole kernel, solids & liq.	4¼ oz.	16.7
Whole kernel, *Mexicorn,* solids & liq.	3½ oz.	18.6
(Libby's):		
Cream style	½ cup	21.2

Food and Description	Measure or Quantity	Carbohydrates (grams)
Whole kernel, solids & liq.	½ cup	18.8
(Stokely-Van Camp):		
Cream style	½ cup	23.5
Whole kernel, solids & liq.	½ cup	19.5
Canned, dietetic pack:		
(Diet Delight) solids & liq.	½ cup	15.0
(Featherweight) whole kernel, solids & liq.	½ cup	16.0
(S&W) *Nutradiet*, solids & liq.	½ cup	15.0
Frozen:		
(Birds Eye):		
On the cob:		
Farmside	4.4-oz. ear	28.7
Little Ears	2.3-oz. ear	.6
Whole kernel	⅓ of pkg.	19.4
(Green Giant):		
On the cob	5½" ear	27.4
On the cob, *Nibbler*	3" ear	15.1
Whole kernel, *Harvest Fresh*	4 oz.	21.9
Whole kernel, *Niblets*, golden, in butter sauce	⅓ of pkg.	15.2
Whole kernel, white, in butter sauce	⅓ of pkg.	15.9
(McKenzie) on the cob	5" ear	29.0
(Seabrook Farms):		
On the cob	5" ear	30.0
Whole kernel	⅓ of pkg.	19.9
CORNBREAD:		
Home recipe:		
Corn pone	4 oz.	41.1
Spoon bread	4 oz.	19.2
*Mix:		
(Aunt Jemima)	⅙ of pkg.	34.0
(Dromedary)	2" × 2" piece	19.0
(Pillsbury) *Ballard*	⅛ of recipe	25.0
*CORN DOGS, frozen (Oscar Mayer)	4-oz. piece	27.9
CORNED BEEF:		
Cooked, boneless, medium fat	4 oz.	0.
Canned:		
Dinty Moore	3-oz. serving	0.
(Libby's)	⅓ of 7-oz. can	2.0
Packaged:		
(Eckrich) sliced	1-oz. slice	.9
(Oscar Mayer) jellied loaf	1-oz. slice	0.
(Vienna):		
Brisket	1-oz. serving	0.

Food and Description	Measure or Quantity	Carbohydrates (grams)
Flats	1-oz. serving	.1
(Libby's)	1 cup	21.0
Mary Kitchen	7½-oz. serving	21.1
CORNED BEEF HASH DINNER, frozen (Banquet)	10-oz.dinner	42.6
CORNED BEEF SPREAD (Underwood)	1 oz.	Tr.
CORN FLAKE CRUMBS (Kellogg's)	¼ cup	25.0
CORN FLAKES, (cereal):		
(Featherweight) low sodium	1¼ cups	25.0
(General Mills) *Country*	1 cup	25.0
(Kellogg's)	1 cup	25.0
(Kellogg's) honey & nut	¾ cup	24.0
(Post) *Post Toasties*	1¼ cups	24.4
(Ralston Purina) regular	1 cup	25.0
(Van Brode)	1 oz.	24.3
CORN MEAL:		
Bolted (Aunt Jemima/Quaker)	3 T.	22.0
Degermed	¼ cup	27.0
Mix Bolted (Aunt Jemima)	1 cup	124.8
CORNNUTS	1-oz. serving	21.0
CORNSTARCH (Argo: Kingsford's; Duryea)	1 tsp.	2.8
CORN SYRUP (See SYRUP)		
COUGH DROP:		
(Beech-Nut)	1 drop	2.5
(Pine Bros.)	1 drop	2.0
COUNT CHOCULA, cereal (General Mills)	1 oz. (1 cup)	24.0
CRAB:		
Fresh,steamed:		
Whole	½ lb.	.6
Meat only	4 oz.	.6
Canned, king crab (Icy Point; Pillar Rock)	3¾ oz.	1.6
Frozen (Wakefield's Alaska King)	4 oz.	.7
CRAB APPLE, flesh only	¼ lb.	20.2
CRAB APPLE JELLY (Smucker's)	1 T.	13.5
CRAB, DEVILED, breaded & fried (Mrs. Paul's) regular	½ of 6-oz. pkg.	17.0
CRAB IMPERIAL, home recipe	1 cup	8.6
CRACKER, PUFFS & CHIPS:		
Arrowroot biscuit (Nabisco)	1 piece	3.5
Bacon'n Dip (Nabisco)	1 piece	.9
Bacon-flavored thins (Nabisco)	1 piece	1.2.
Bacon Nips	1 oz.	15.6

Food and Description	Measure or Quantity	Carbohydrates (grams)
Bacon Toast (Keebler)	1 piece	2.0
Biscos (Nabisco)	1 piece	2.6
Bran Wafer (Featherweight)	1 piece	2.0
Bugles (General Mills)	1 oz.	18.0
Cheese flavored:		
Cheddar triangles (Nabisco)	1 piece	.9
Cheese'n Crunch (Nabisco)	1 oz.	14.0
Chee-Tos, crunchy	1 oz.	15.0
Chee-Tos, puffed	1 oz.	15.0
Cheez Balls (Planters)	1 oz.	15.0
Cheez Curls (Planters)	1 oz.	15.0
Country cheddar'n sesame (Nabisco)	1 piece	1.0
Nacho cheese cracker (Keebler)	1 piece	1.6
Nips (Nabisco)	1 piece	.7
Ralston)	1 piece	.7
Swiss cheese (Nabisco)	1 piece	1.1
Tid-Bit (Nabisco)	1 oz.	.5
Twists (Bachman) baked	1 oz.	17.0
Chicken in a Biskit (Nabisco)	1 piece	1.1
Chip O'Cheddar, Flavor Kist, (Schulze and Burch)	1 oz.	17.0
Chippers (Nabisco)	1 piece	1.7
Club cracker (Keebler)	1 piece	2.1
Corn chips:		
(Bachman) regular or bag	1 oz.	15.0
(Featherweight)	1 oz.	15.0
Fritos, regular or barbecue	1 oz.	16.0
Corn Nuts (Nalley's)	1 oz.	20.4
Corn & Sesame Chips (Nabisco)	1 piece	.9
Creme Wafer Stock (Nabisco)	1 piece	6.3
Crown Pilot (Nabisco)	1 piece	13.0
Dixies (Nabisco)	1 piece	.9
English Water Biscuit (Pepperidge Farm)	1 piece	3.1
Escort (Nabisco)	1 piece	2.6
Flings (Nabisco)	1 piece	.9
Goldfish (Pepperidge Farm):		
Thins	1 piece	1.1
Tiny	1 piece	.4
Graham:		
(Dixie Belle) Sugar-honey coated	1 piece	2.6
Flavor Kist (Schulze and Burch) sugar-honey coated	1 piece	10.0
Honey Maid (Nabisco)	1 piece	5.5

Food and Description	Measure or Quantity	Carbohydrates (grams)
Graham, chocolate or cocoa-covered:		
Fancy Dip (Nabisco)	1 piece	8.0
(Keebler)	1 piece	5.6
(Nabisco)	1 piece	7.0
Melba Toast (See MELBA TOAST)		
Muncho Macho Nacho, Flavor Kist,		
(Schulze and Burch)	1 oz.	18.0
Onion Toast (Keebler)	1 piece	2.1
Oyster:		
(Keebler) *Zesta*	1 piece	.3
(Nabisco) *Dandy* or *Oysterettes*	1 piece	.5
Pumpernickel Toast (Keebler)	1 piece	2.1
Ritz (Nabisco)	1 piece	2.0
Roman Meal Wafer, boxed	1 piece	1.3
Royal Lunch (Nabisco)	1 piece	8.0
Rusk, *Holland* (Nabisco)	1 piece	7.5
Rye Toast (Keebler)	1 piece	2.1
Ry-Krisp, natural or sesame	1 triple cracker	5.0
Ry-Krisp, seasoned	1 triple cracker	4.5
Saltine:		
(Dixie Belle) regular or unsalted	1 piece	2.1
Flavor Kist (Schulze and Burch)	1 piece	2.0
Premium (Nabisco)	1 piece	2.0
Zesta (Keebler)	1 piece	2.1
Sesame:		
Butter flavored (Nabisco)	1 piece	1.9
Sesame Wheats! (Nabisco)	1 piece	1.8
Sesame wheat snack, *Flavor Kist*		
(Schulze and Burch)	1 oz.	18.0
Sticks (Keebler)	1 piece	.8
Teeko (Nabisco)	1 piece	3.0
Toast (Keebler)	1 piece	
Shindigs (Keebler)	1 piece	.9
Snackers (Ralston)	1 piece	Tr.
Snackin' Crisp (Durkee) *O & C*	1 oz.	15.0
Snacks Sticks (Pepperidge Farm):		
Lightly salted, pumpernickel or rye	1 piece	2.5
Sesame	1 oz.	2.3
Sociables (Nabisco)	1 piece	1.3
Table Water Cracker (Carr's) small	1 piece	2.5
Tater Puffs (Nabisco)	1 piece	
Tortilla chips:		
(Bachman) nacho, taco flavor or		
toasted	1 oz.	17.0
Buenos (Nabisco) nacho or taco		
flavor	1 piece	1.2

Food and Description	Measure or Quantity	Carbohydrates (grams)
Doritos, nacho or taco flavor	1 oz.	18.0
Tostitos	1 oz.	17.0
Town House Cracker (Keebler)	1 piece	1.8
Triscuit (Nabisco)	1 piece	3.0
Uneeda Biscuit (Nabisco)	1 piece	3.7
Unsalted (Featherweight)	2 sections (½ cracker)	5.0
Vegetable thins (Nabisco)	1 piece	1.3
Waldorf (Keebler)	1 piece	2.3
Waverly Wafer (Nabisco)	1 piece	2.6
Wheat (Pepperidge Farm) cracked or hearty	1 piece	3.8
Wheat Chips (Nabisco)	1 piece	.5
Wheatmeal Biscuit (Carr's) small	1 piece	5.9
Wheat snack, *Flavor Kist* (Schulze and Burch):		
Regular	1 oz.	16.0
Wild onion	1 oz.	18.0
Wheat Snack (Ralston)	1 piece	1.2
Wheatsworth (Nabisco)	1 piece	1.8
Wheat Thins (Nabisco)	1 piece	1.2
CRACKER CRUMBS, graham (Nabisco)	⅛ of 9″ pie shell	12.0
CRACKER MEAL (Nabisco)	½ cup	47.5
CRANAPPLE JUICE (Ocean Spray) canned:		
Regular	6 fl. oz.	32.1
Dietetic	6 fl. oz.	7.4
CRANBERRY, fresh (Ocean Spray)	½ cup	6.1
*CRANBERRY-APPLE JUICE, frozen (Welch's)	6 fl. oz.	30.0
*CRANBERRY-GRAPE JUICE, frozen (Welch's)	6 fl. oz.	27.0
*CRANBERRY JUICE COCKTAIL:		
Canned (Ocean Spray):		
Regular	6 fl. oz.	26.4
Dietetic	6 fl. oz.	8.3
*Frozen (Welch's)	6 fl. oz.	26.0
CRANBERRY-ORANGE RELISH (Ocean Spray)	1 T.	25.8
CRANBERRY-RASPBERRY SAUCE (Ocean Spray) jellied	2-oz. serving	20.8
CRANBERRY SAUCE:		
Home recipe	4 oz.	51.6
Canned (Ocean Spray):		
Jellied	2-oz. serving	21.7

Food and Description	Measure or Quantity	Carbohydrates (grams)
Whole berry	2-oz. serving	22.0
CRANGRAPE (Ocean Spray)	6 fl. oz.	26.3
CRANICOT (Ocean Spray)	6 fl. oz.	30.4
CRAZY COW, cereal (General Mills)	1 cup	25.0
CREAM:		
Half & Half (Dairylea)	1 fl. oz.	1.0
Light, table or coffee (Sealtest) 16% fat	1 T.	.6
Light, whipping, 30% fat (Sealtest)	1 T.	1.0
Heavy whipping (Dairylea)	1 fl. oz.	1.0
Sour (Dairylea)	1 fl. oz.	1.0
Sour, imitation (Pet)	1 T.	1.0
Substitute (See CREAM SUBSTITUTE)		
CREAM PUFFS:		
Home recipe, custard filling	3½" × 2" piece	26.7
Frozen (Rich's) chocolate	1⅓ oz. piece	16.9
CREAMSICLE (Popsicle Industries)	2½-fl.-oz. piece	13.0
CREAM SUBSTITUTE:		
Coffee Mate (Carnation)	.1-oz. packet	1.6
Coffee Rich	½ oz.	2.1
Dairy Light (Alba)	2.8-oz. envelope	1.0
N-Rich	1½ tsp.	1.6
CREAM OF WHEAT, cereal:		
*Instant	1 T.	8.8
Mix'n Eat, dry:		
Regular	1 packet	24.0
Baked apple & cinnamon or maple & brown sugar	1 packet	32.0
Quick	2½ T.	22.0
Regular	2½ T.	22.0
CREME DE BANANA LIQUEUR (Mr. Boston)	1 fl. oz.	12.0
CREME DE CACAO:		
(Garnier)	1 fl. oz.	13.1
(Hiram Walker)	1 fl. oz.	15.0
(Mr. Boston):		
Brown	1 fl. oz.	14.3
White	1 fl. oz.	12.0
CREME DE CASSIS:		
(Garnier)	1 fl. oz.	13.5
(Mr. Boston)	1 fl. oz.	14.1
CREME DE MENTHE:		
(Hiram Walker)	1 fl. oz.	11.2
(Mr. Boston):		
Green	1 fl. oz.	16.0

Food and Description	Measure or Quantity	Carbohydrates (grams)
White	1 fl. oz.	13.0
CREME DE NOYAUX (Mr. Boston)	1 fl. oz.	13.5
CREPE, frozen:		
(Mrs. Paul's):		
Crab	5½-oz. pkg.	24.6
Shrimp	5½-oz. pkg.	23.8
(Stouffer's):		
Beef burgundy	6¼-oz. pkg.	24.0
Chicken with mushroom sauce	8¼-oz. pkg.	19.0
Ham & asparagus	6¼-oz. pkg.	21.0
Mushroom	6¼-oz. pkg.	27.0
CRISP RICE, cereal:		
(Featherweight) low sodium	1 cup	26.0
(Ralston Purina)	1 cup	25.0
(Van Brode) regular	1 cup	24.9
CRISPY WHEATS'N RAISINS, cereal		
(General Mills)	¾ cup	23.0
CROQUETTES, frozen, seafood		
(Mrs. Paul's)	3-oz. serving	23.9
CROUTON:		
(Arnold):		
Bavarian or English style	½ oz.	9.5
French, Italian or Mexican style	½ oz.	9.2
(Kellogg's) *Croutettes*	⅔ cup	14.0
(Pepperidge Farm):		
Cheddar and romano or onion and garlic	.5 oz.	10.0
Cheese and garlic or sour cream and chive	.5 oz.	9.0
CUCUMBER:		
Eaten with skin	½-lb. cucumber	7.4
Pared, 10-oz. cucumber	7½″ × 2″ pared	6.6
Pared	3 slices	.8
CUMIN SEED (French's)	1 tsp.	.7
CUPCAKE:		
Regular (Hostess):		
Chocolate	1 cupcake	29.8
Orange	1 cupcake	26.8
Frozen (Sara Lee) yellow	1 cupcake	31.5
***CUPCAKE MIX** (Flako)	1 cupcake	25.0
CUP O'NOODLES (Nissin Foods):		
Beef	2½-oz. serving	39.2
Beef, twin pack	1.2-oz. serving	18.2
Beef onion	2½-oz. serving	36.8
Beef onion, twin pack	1.2-oz. serving	19.4
Chicken	2½-oz. serving	40.0

Food and Description	Measure or Quantity	Carbohydrates (grams)
Chicken, twin pack	1.2-oz. serving	18.6
Pork	2½-oz. serving	40.7
Shrimp	2½-oz. serving	40.0
CURACAO:		
(Bols)	1 fl. oz.	10.3
(Hiram Walker)	1 fl. oz.	11.8
CURRANT, dried, Zante (Del Monte)	½ cup	47.8
CURRANT JELLY (Smucker's)	1 T.	13.5
C.W. POST, cereal, plain or raisin	¼ cup	20.4

D

Food and Description	Measure or Quantity	Carbohydrates (grams)
DAIRY QUEEN/BRAZIER:		
Banana split	13.5-oz. serving	103.0
Brownie Delight, hot fudge	9.4-oz. serving	85.0
Buster Bar	5¼-oz. piece	41.0
Chicken sandwich	7.76-oz. sandwich	46.0
Cone:		
Plain, any flavor:		
Small	3-oz. cone	22.0
Regular	5-oz. cone	38.0
Large	7½-oz. cone	57.0
Dipped, chocolate:		
Small	3¼-oz. cone	25.0
Regular	5½-oz. cone	42.0
Large	8¼-oz. cone	64.0
Dilly Bar	3-oz. piece	21.0
Double Delight	9-oz. serving	69.0
DO sandwich	2.1-oz. serving	24.0
Fish sandwich:		
Plain	6-oz. sandwich	41.0
With cheese	6.24-oz. sandwich	39.0
Float	14-oz. serving	82.0
Freeze, vanilla	14-oz. serving	89.0
French fries:		
Regular	2½-oz. serving	25.0
Large	4-oz. serving	40.0
Frozen dessert	4-oz. serving	27.0
Hamburger:		
Plain	Any size	33.0
With cheese:		
Single	5.7-oz. sandwich	33.0
Double	8.43-oz. sandwich	34.0
Triple	10.62-oz. sandwich	34.0

Food and Description	Measure or Quantity	Carbohydrates (grams)
Hot dog:		
Regular:		
Plain	3.53-oz. serving	21.0
With cheese	4-oz. serving	21.0
With chili	4½-oz. serving	23.0
Super:		
Plain	6.2-oz. serving	44.0
With cheese	6.9-oz. serving	45.0
With chili	7.7.-oz. serving	47.0
Lettuce	½ oz.	< 1.0
Malt, chocolate:		
Small	10.26-oz. serving	91.0
Regular	14.74-oz. serving	134.0
Large	20.74-oz. serving	187.0
Mr. Misty:		
Plain:		
Small	8¾-oz. serving	48.0
Regular	11.64-oz. serving	63.0
Large	15.5-oz. serving	84.0
Kiss	3.14-oz. serving	17.0
Float	14½-oz. serving	74.0
Freeze	14½-oz. serving	94.0
Onion rings	3-oz.	31.0
Parfait	10 oz.	76.0
Peanut Butter Parfait	10¾-oz. serving	94.0
Shake: chocolate:		
Small	10¼-oz. serving	82.0
Regular	14¾-oz. serving	120.0
Large	20¾-oz. serving	168.0
Strawberry shortcake	11 oz.	100.0
Sundae, chocolate:		
Small	3¾-oz. serving	33.0
Regular	6¼-oz. serving	56.0
Large	8¾-oz. serving	78.0
Tomato	½ oz.	1.0
DAIQUIRI COCKTAIL, canned (Mr. Boston):		
Regular	3 fl. oz.	9.0
Strawberry	3 fl. oz.	12.0
DATE (Dromedary):		
Chopped	¼ cup	31.0
Pitted	5 dates	23.0
DELI'S, frozen (Pepperidge Farm):		
Beef with barbecue sauce	4 oz.	30.0
Reuben in rye pastry	4 oz.	25.0
Savory chicken salad	4 oz.	26.0

Food and Description	Measure or Quantity	Carbohydrates (grams)
Turkey, ham and cheese	4 oz.	24.0
Western style omelet	4 oz.	27.0
DESSERT CUPS (Hostess)	¾-oz. piece	13.8
DILL SEED (French's)	1 tsp.	1.2
DING DONG (Hostess)	1 cake	21.5
DINNER, frozen (See individual listings such as BEEF, CHICKEN, TURKEY, etc.)		
DIP:		
Avocado (Nalley's)	1 oz.	.9
Barbecue (Nalley's)	1 oz.	1.1
Blue cheese:		
(Dean) tang	1 oz.	2.3
(Nalley's)	1 oz.	.9
Clam (Nalley's)	1 oz.	1.1
Enchilada, *Fritos*	1 oz.	3.9
Garlic (Nalley's)	1 oz.	.9
Guacamole (Nalley's)	1 oz.	.9
Jalapeno:		
Fritos	1 oz.	3.7
(Hain) natural	1 oz.	2.5
Onion (Dean) French	1 oz.	1.9
Onion bean (Hain) natural	1 oz.	3.6
DISTILLED LIQUOR, any brand, any proof	1 fl. oz.	Tr.
DONUTZ, cereal (General Mills)	1 cup	23.0
DOUGHNUT (See also *Winchell's):*		
Regular (Hostess):		
Chocolate covered	1-oz. piece	13.6
Crunch	1-oz. piece	16.5
Donettes, frosted or powdered	1 piece	6.0
Old fashioned, plain	1½-oz. piece	30.7
Powdered	1-oz. piece	15.1
Frozen (Morton):		
Boston creme	2.3-oz. piece	28.5
Chocolate iced	1½-oz. piece	19.6
Jelly	1.8-oz. piece	22.9
DRAMBUIE (Hiram Walker)	1 fl. oz.	11.0
DRUMSTICK, frozen:		
Ice cream, in a cone:		
Topped with peanuts	1 piece	22.7
Topped with peanuts, and cone bisque	1 piece	23.6
Ice milk, in a cone:		
Topped with peanuts	1 piece	24.3

Food and Description	Measure or Quantity	Carbohydrates (grams)
Topped with peanuts and cone bisque	1 piece	25.2
DUMPLINGS, canned, dietetic (Featherweight)	7½ oz.	18.0

E

Food and Description	Measure or Quantity	Carbohydrates (grams)
ECLAIR:		
Home recipe, with custard filling and chocolate icing	4-oz. piece	26.3
Frozen (Rich's) chocolate	1 piece	30.0
EGG, CHICKEN:		
Raw, white only	1 large egg	.3
Boiled	1 large egg	.4
Fried in butter	1 large egg	.1
Omelet, mixed with milk and cooked in fat	1 large egg	1.5
Poached	1 large egg	.4
Scrambled, mixed with milk and cooked in fat	1 large egg	1.5
***EGG FOO YOUNG** (Chun King) stir fry	⅙ of pkg.	3.0
EGG MIX (Durkee):		
Omelet:		
*With bacon	½ of pkg.	10.0
*Puffy	½ of pkg.	10.5
Scrambled:		
Plain	.8-oz. pkg.	4.0
With bacon	1.3-oz. pkg.	6.0
EGG NOG, dairy (Meadow Gold) 6% fat	½ cup	25.5
EGG NOG COCKTAIL (Mr. Boston) 15% alcohol	3 fl. oz.	18.9
EGGPLANT:		
Frozen:		
(Mrs. Paul's):		
Parmesan	5½-oz. serving	21.6
Slices, breaded and fried	3-oz. serving	22.4
Sticks, breaded and fried	3½-oz. serving	27.3
(Weight Watchers) parmigiana	13-oz. pkg.	25.0
EGG ROLL: frozen:		
(Chun King):		
Chicken	½-oz. roll	3.0
Shrimp	½-oz. roll	3.8

Food and Description	Measure or Quantity	Carbohydrates (grams)
(La Choy):		
Chicken or lobster	.4-oz. roll	3.6
Meat and shrimp	.2-oz. roll	2.3
Shrimp	2½-oz. roll	14.9
EGG, SCRAMBLED, frozen (Swanson) and sausage with hashed brown potatoes, TV Brand	6½-oz. entree	17.0
EGG SUBSTITUTE:		
Egg Magic (Featherweight)	½ envelope	1.0
Eggstra (Tillie Lewis) *Tasti-Diet*	1 egg	4.0
Scramblers (Morningstar Farms)	1 egg	1.2
Second Nature (Avoset)	3 T.	2.0
ELDERBERRY JELLY (Smucker's)	1 T.	13.5
ENCHILADA, frozen:		
Beef:		
(Banquet):		
Buffet Supper, with cheese and chili gravy	2-lb. pkg.	118.2
Dinner	12-oz. dinner	63.6
(Green Giant) Sonora style	12-oz. entree	47.7
(Swanson) *TV Brand*	15-oz. dinner	72.0
(Van de Kamp's):		
Dinner	12-oz. dinner	45.0
Entree, shredded	12-oz. entree	40.0
Cheese:		
(Banquet) *Man-Pleaser*	21¼-oz. dinner	82.0
(Van de Kamp's)	12-oz. dinner	44.0
Chicken (Van de Kamp's)	7½-oz. pkg.	24.0
ENCHILADA SAUCE:		
Canned (Del Monte) hot or mild	½ cup	11.0
*Mix (Durkee)	½ cup	6.2
ENDIVE, CURLY OR ESCAROLE, cut up	½ cup	1.4
EXPRESSO COFFEE LIQUEUR	1 fl. oz.	15.0

F

FARINA:		
(Hi-O) dry, regular	¼ cup	33.6
Malt-O-Meal, dry, regular	1 oz.	21.0
Malt-O-Meal, dry, quick cooking	1 oz.	22.2
*(Pillsbury) made with milk and salt	⅔ cup	17.0
FAT, COOKING	1 T.	0
FENNEL SEED (French's)	1 tsp.	1.3

Food and Description	Measure or Quantity	Carbohydrates (grams)
FIG:		
Small	1½" fig	7.7
Canned, regular pack (Del Monte) whole, solids & liq.	½ cup	27.7
Dried, chopped	½ cup	59.1
FIG JUICE, *RealFig*	½ cup	15.8
FIGURINES (Pillsbury) all flavors	1 bar	10.5
FILBERT:		
Shelled	1 oz.	14.7
(Fisher) oil dipped, salted	½ cup	5.4
FISH CAKE, frozen (Mrs. Paul's):		
Breaded and fried	2-oz. cake	11.9
Thins, breaded and fried	½ of 10-oz. pkg.	30.7
FISH & CHIPS, frozen:		
(Mrs. Paul's) batter fried, light	½ of 14-oz. pkg.	43.3
(Swanson) *TV Brand*	5-oz. entree	30.0
(Van de Kamp's) batter dipped, french fried	8-oz. serving	45.0
FISH DINNER, frozen:		
(Banquet)	8¾-oz. dinner	43.6
(Mrs. Paul's):		
Au gratin	½ of 10-oz. pkg.	19.6
Parmesan	½ of 10-oz. pkg.	20.9
(Van de Kamp's) batter dipped, french fried	11-oz. dinner	39.0
(Weight Watchers) in lemon sauce, 3-compartment	13¼-oz. meal	19.1
FISH FILLET, frozen:		
(Mrs. Paul's):		
Batter fried, crunchy	2¼-oz. piece	17.2
Breaded and fried	2-oz. piece	12.0
Miniature, batter fried	3-oz. serving	15.3
(Van de Kamp's):		
Batter dipped, french fried	3-oz. piece	12.5
Country seasoned	2.4-oz. piece	10.5
FISH KABOBS, frozen:		
(Mrs. Paul's) light batter	⅓ pkg.	17.7
(Van de Kamp's):		
Batter dipped	.4-oz. piece	1.6
Country seasoned	.4-oz. piece	1.9
FISH SANDWICH, frozen,		
(Mrs. Paul's) fillet	4⅛-oz. sandwich	23.2
FISH SEASONING (Featherweight)	¼ tsp.	Tr.
FISH STICK, frozen:		
(Mrs. Paul's):		
Batter fried	1 stick	6.4

Food and Description	Measure or Quantity	Carbohydrates (grams)
Breaded and fried	1 stick	4.1
(Van de Kamp's) batter dipped, french fried	1-oz. piece	5.2
FIT 'N FROSTY (Alba '77):		
Chocolate or marshmallow flavor	1 envelope	11.0
Strawberry	1 envelope	12.0
Vanilla	1 envelope	11.3
***FIVE ALIVE** (Snow Crop)	6 fl. oz.	20.8
FLOUNDER:		
Baked	4 oz.	0.
Frozen:		
(Mrs. Paul's) fillets, breaded & fried	2-oz. fillet	11.6
(Mrs. Paul's) with lemon butter	4¼-oz. serving	9.4
(Weight Watchers) with lemon flavored bread crumbs	6½-oz. serving	12.0
(Weight Watchers) in Newburgh sauce	12½-oz. pkg.	11.0
FLOUR:		
(Aunt Jemima) self-rising	¼ cup	23.6
Ballard, self-rising	¼ cup	21.3
Bisquick (Betty Crocker)	¼ cup	19.0
(Elam's):		
Brown rice, whole grain	¼ cup	30.1
Buckwheat, pure	¼ cup	19.0
Pastry	1 oz.	20.7
Rye, whole grain	¼ cup	18.2
Soy	1 oz.	8.9
Gold Medal (Betty Crocker) all-purpose or high protein	¼ cup	21.8
La Pina	¼ cup	21.6
Pillsbury's Best:		
All-purpose	¼ cup	21.5
Rye, medium	¼ cup	20.8
Sauce and gravy	2 T.	11.0
Self-rising	¼ cup	21.0
Presto, self-rising	¼ cup	21.6
Wondra	¼ cup	21.8
FOOD STICKS (Pillsbury)		
Chocolate	1 stick	6.8
FRANKEN*BERRY, cereal (General Mills)	1 cup	24.0
FRANKFURTER:		
(Best's Kosher):		
Regular	1.5-oz. frankfurter	1.5
Beef	1.5-oz. frankfurter	1.5

Food and Description	Measure or Quantity	Carbohydrates (grams)
Dinner	2.7-oz. frankfurter	2.7
(Eckrich):		
Beef or meat	1.6-oz. frankfurter	3.0
Beef or meat, jumbo	2-oz. frankfurter	3.0
Meat	1.2-oz. frankfurter	2.0
(Hormel):		
Beef	1.6-oz. frankfurter	.7
Range Brand, Wrangler, smoked	1 frankfurter	2.0
(Hygrade) Beef, Ball Park	2-oz. frankfurter	<1.0
(Louis Rich) Turkey	1.5-oz. frankfurter	1.0
(Oscar Mayer):		
Beef	1.6-oz. frankfurter	.9
Little Wiener	2″ frankfurter	.2
Wiener	1.6-oz. frankfurter	.8
Wiener, with cheese	1.6-oz. frankfurter	.7
(Oscherwitz):		
Regular	1.6-oz. frankfurter	1.6
Cocktail	.3-oz. frankfurter	.3
(Vienna) beef	1.5-oz. frankfurter	1.0
FRANKS-N-BLANKETS (Durkee)	1 piece	1.0
FRENCH TOAST, frozen:		
(Aunt Jemima):		
Regular	1½-oz. slice	13.2
Cinnamon swirl	1 slice	13.6
(Swanson) with sausage, *TV Brand*	4½-oz. breakfast	28.0
FRITTERS, frozen (Mrs. Paul's):		
Apple	2-oz. piece	16.1
Clam	1.9-oz. piece	14.3
Corn	2-oz. piece	1.1
Shrimp	½ of 7¾-oz. pkg.	27.0
FROOT LOOPS, cereal (Kellogg's)	1 cup	25.0
FROSTED RICE, cereal (Kellogg's)	1 cup	26.0
FROSTS (Libby's):		
Dry, all flavors	.5 oz.	14.0
Liquid:		
Banana	7 fl. oz.	25.0
Orange	8 fl. oz.	29.0
Pineapple	6 fl. oz.	22.0
FROZEN DESSERT dietetic:		
Good Humor:		
Bar, vanilla with chocolate coating	2½-oz. bar	12.0
Cup, vanilla and chocolate	5-fl.-oz. cup	17.0
(SugarLo) all flavors	¼ pt.	14.0

Food and Description	Measure or Quantity	Carbohydrates (grams)
FRUIT COCKTAIL:		
Canned, regular pack, solids & liq.:		
(Del Monte) regular and chunky	½ cup	22.8
(Libby's)	½ cup	24.7
(Stokely-Van Camp)	½ cup	23.0
Canned, dietetic pack, solids & liq.:		
(Del Monte) *Lite*	½ cup	14.1
(Diet Delight):		
Syrup pack	½ cup	14.0
Water pack	½ cup	10.0
(Featherweight):		
Juice pack	½ cup	12.0
Water pack	½ cup	10.0
(Libby's) water pack	½ cup	13.0
(S&W) *Nutradiet:*		
Juice pack	½ cup	14.0
Water pack	½ cup	10.0
***FRUIT COUNTRY** (Comstock):*		
Apple	¼ of pkg.	36.0
Blueberry	¼ of pkg.	33.0
Cherry	¼ of pkg.	38.0
FRUIT CUP (Del Monte):		
Mixed fruits	5-oz. container	26.7
Peaches, diced	5-oz. container	27.8
***FRUIT AND FIBER,** cereal (Post)*	½ cup	22.3
FRUIT JUICE, canned (Sun-Maid)	6 fl. oz.	23.0
FRUIT, MIXED:		
Canned (Del Monte) *Lite*	½ cup	13.6
Frozen (Birds Eye) quick thaw	5-oz. serving	35.8
FRUIT PUNCH:		
Canned:		
Capri Sun	6¾ fl. oz.	25.9
(Hi-C)	6 fl. oz.	23.0
(Lincoln) party	6 fl. oz.	25.0
Chilled:		
Five Alive (Snow Crop)	6 fl. oz.	22.7
(Minute Maid)	6 fl. oz.	23.0
*Frozen, *Five Alive* (Snow Crop)	6 fl. oz.	22.7
*Mix (Hi-C)	6 fl. oz.	18.0
FRUIT ROLL, frozen (La Choy)	.5-oz. roll	6.4
***FRUIT ROLL-UPS,** (Betty Crocker)*	1 roll	12.0
FRUIT SALAD:		
Canned, regular pack:		
(Del Monte) fruits for salad	½ cup	22.6
(Libby's)	½ cup	24.0

Food and Description	Measure or Quantity	Carbohydrates (grams)
Canned, dietetic pack:		
(Diet Delight)	½ cup	16.0
(Featherweight):		
Juice pack	½ cup	12.0
(S&W) *Nutradiet:*		
Juice pack	½ cup	14.0
Water pack	½ cup	10.0
FRUIT SQUARES, frozen		
(Pepperidge Farm):		
Apple	2½-oz. piece	27.0
Blueberry or cherry	2½-oz. piece	29.0
FUDGESICLE (Popsicle Industries)	2½-fl.-oz. bar	23.0

G

Food and Description	Measure or Quantity	Carbohydrates (grams)
GARLIC:		
Flakes (Gilroy)	1 tsp.	2.6
Powder (French's)	1 tsp.	2.0
Salt (French's)	1 tsp.	1.0
GELFILTE FISH, canned:		
(Mother's):		
Jelled, old world	4-oz. serving	7.0
Jelled, Whitefish and Pike	4-oz. serving	4.0
In liquid broth	4-oz. serving	7.0
(Rokeach):		
Jelled, Whitefish and Pike	4-oz. serving	4.0
Old Vienna	4-oz. serving	8.0
GELATIN, dry, *Carmel Kosher*	7-gram envelope	0.
GELATIN DESSERT MIX:		
Regular:		
Carmel Kosher, all flavors	½ cup	20.0
(Jell-O)	½ cup	18.7
Dietetic:		
Carmel Kosher	½ cup	0.
(D-ZERTA)	½ cup	Tr.
(Estee) all flavors	½ cup	9.9
(Featherweight) artificially sweetened	½ cup	0.
GELATIN, DRINKING (Knox) orange	1 envelope	10.0
GERMAN STYLE DINNER (Swanson) *TV Brand*	11¾-oz. dinner	36.0
GINGER, powder (French's)	1 tsp.	1.2
***GINGERBREAD MIX:**		
(Betty Crocker)	⅑ of cake	35.0

Food and Description	Measure or Quantity	Carbohydrates (grams)
(Dromedary)	2″ × 2″ square	20.0
(Pillsbury)	3″ square	26.0
GIN, SLOE:		
(DeKuyper)	1 fl. oz.	5.2
(Hiram Walker)	1 fl. oz.	4.8
(Mr. Boston)	1 fl. oz.	4.7
GOLDEN GRAHAMS, cereal		
(General Mills)	¾ cup	24.0
GOOBER GRAPE (Smucker's)	1 oz.	14.0
GOOD HUMOR (See ICE CREAM)		
GOOD N' PUDDIN (Popsicle Industries) all flavors	2¼-fl.-oz. bar	27.0
GOOSE, roasted, meat and skin	4 oz.	0.
GRAHAM CRAKOS, cereal		
(Kellogg's)	1 cup	24.0
GRANOLA BARS, *Nature Valley:*		
Almond, cinnamon or oats'n honey	1 bar (.8 oz.)	16.0
Coconut or peanut	1 bar	15.0
GRANOLA BAR MIX, chewy		
(Nature Valley)	1 bar	16.0
GRANOLA CEREAL:		
Nature Valley:		
Cinnamon and raisin or fruit and nut	⅓ cup	19.0
Coconut and honey	⅓ cup	18.0
Sun Country:		
With almonds	½ cup	34.1
With raisins	½ cup	36.9
GRANOLA CLUSTERS, *Nature Valley:*		
Almond	1 roll	27.0
Apple cinnamon	1 roll	25.0
Caramel or raisin	1 roll	28.0
GRANOLA AND FRUIT BAR, *Nature Valley*	1 bar	25.0
GRAPE:		
American ripe (slipskin)	3½″ × 3″ bunch	9.9
Canned, dietetic (Featherweight) light, seedless, water pack	½ cup	13.0
GRAPE DRINK:		
Canned:		
Capri Sun	6¾ fl. oz.	26.3
(Hi-C)	6 fl. oz.	22.0
Lincoln)	6 fl. oz.	23.9
(Welchade)	6 fl. oz.	23.0

Food and Description	Measure or Quantity	Carbohydrates (grams)
*Frozen (Welchade)	6 fl. oz.	23.0
*Mix (Hi-C)	6 fl. oz.	17.0
GRAPEFRUIT:		
Pink and red:		
Seeded type	½ med. grapefruit	11.9
Seedless type	½ med. grapefruit	12.8
White:		
Seeded type	½ med. grapefruit	11.7
Seedless type	½ med. grapefruit	11.9
Canned, regular pack (Del Monte) in syrup	½ cup	17.5
Canned, dietetic pack, solids and liq.:		
(Del Monte) sections	½ cup	10.4
(Diet Delight) sections	½ cup	11.0
(Featherweight) sections, juice pack	½ cup	9.0
GRAPEFRUIT DRINK, canned (Lincoln)	6 fl. oz.	25.0
GRAPEFRUIT JUICE:		
Fresh, pick, red or white	½ cup	11.3
Canned, sweetened:		
(Del Monte)	6 fl. oz.	20.8
(Minute Maid)	6 fl. oz.	17.0
Canned, unsweetened:		
(Del Monte)	6 fl. oz.	16.6
(Libby's)	6 fl. oz.	18.0
(Ocean Spray)	6 fl. oz.	14.5
(Texsun)	6 fl. oz.	18.0
Chilled (Minute Maid)	6 fl. oz.	18.1
*Frozen (Minute Maid)	6 fl. oz.	18.3
GRAPEFRUIT JUICE COCKTAIL, canned (Ocean Spray) pink	6 fl. oz.	20.0
GRAPEFRUIT-ORANGE JUICE COCKTAIL, canned, *Musselman's*	6 fl. oz.	17.2
GRAPE JAM (Smucker's)	1 T.	13.7
GRAPE JELLY:		
Sweetened:		
(Smucker's)	1 T.	13.5
(Welch's)	1 T.	13.5
Dietetic (*See* GRAPE SPREAD)		
GRAPE JUICE:		
Canned, unsweetened:		
(Seneca Foods)	6 fl. oz.	30.0
(Welch's)	6 fl. oz.	30.0

Food and Description	Measure or Quantity	Carbohydrates (grams)
*Frozen:		
(Minute Maid)	6 fl. oz.	13.3
(Welch's)	6 fl. oz.	25.0
GRAPE JUICE DRINK, chilled		
(Welch's)	6 fl. oz.	27.0
GRAPE NUTS, cereal:		
Regular	¼ cup	23.3
Flakes	⅞ cup	23.2
GRAPE SPREAD, dietetic:		
(Diet Delight)	1 T.	3.0
(Estee)	1 T.	1.6
(Featherweight) calorie reduced	1 T.	4.0
(Smucker's)	1 T.	6.0
GRAVY, canned:		
Au jus (Franco-American)	2-oz. serving	2.0
Beef, (Franco-American)	2-oz. serving	3.0
Brown:		
(Franco-American) with onion	2-oz. serving	4.0
(La Choy)	5-oz. can	101.3
Ready Gravy	¼ cup	7.5
Chicken (Franco-American)	2-oz. serving	3.0
Mushroom (Franco-American)	2-oz. serving	3.0
Turkey (Franco-American)	2-oz. serving	3.0
GRAVYMASTER	1 tsp.	2.4
GRAVY WITH MEAT OR TURKEY:		
Canned (Morton House):		
Sliced beef	6¼-oz. serving	8.0
Sliced turkey	6¼-oz. serving	7.0
Frozen:		
(Banquet):		
Giblet gravy, and sliced turkey, *Cookin' Bag*	5-oz. bag	5.3
Sliced beef, *Buffet Supper*	2-lb. pkg.	34.5
(Swanson) sliced beef with whipped potatoes, *TV Brand*	8-oz. entree	19.0
GRAVY MIX:		
Regular:		
Au jus:		
*(Durkee)	½ cup	3.2
*(French's) *Gravy Makins*	½ cup	4.0
Brown:		
*(Durkee):		
Regular	½ cup	5.0
With onions	½ cup	6.5

Food and Description	Measure or Quantity	Carbohydrates (grams)
*(French's) *Gravy Makins*	½ cup	1.5
*(Pillsbury)	½ cup	6.0
*(Spatini)	1-oz. serving	2.0
Chicken:		
(Durkee):		
*Regular	½ cup	7.0
Roastin Bag	1½-oz. pkg.	24.0
*(French's) *Gravy Makins*	½ cup	8.0
*(Pillsbury)	½ cup	8.0
Home style:		
*(Durkee)	½ cup	5.5
*(French's) *Gravy Makins*	½ cup	8.0
*(Pillsbury)	½ cup	6.0
Meatloaf (Durkee) *Roastin' Bag*	1½-oz. pkg.	18.0
Mushroom:		
*(Durkee)	½ cup	5.5
*(French's) *Gravy Makins*	½ cup	6.0
Onion:		
*(Durkee)	½ cup	7.5
*(French's) *Gravy Makins*	½ cup	8.0
Pork:		
*(Durkee)	½ cup	7.0
*(French's) *Gravy Makins*	½ cup	6.0
*Swiss steak (Durkee)	½ cup	5.3
Turkey:		
*(Durkee)	½ cup	7.0
*(French's) *Gravy Makins*	½ cup	8.0
*Dietetic (Weight Watchers):		
Brown	½ cup	2.0
Brown, with mushrooms	½ cup	4.0
Brown, with onion	½ cup	4.0
Chicken	½ cup	4.0
GREENS, MIXED, canned (Sunshine) solids and liq.	½ cup	2.7
GRENADINE (Garnier) no alcohol	1 fl. oz.	26.0
GUAVA NECTAR (Libby's)	6 fl. oz.	17.0

H

HADDOCK:		
Fried, breaded	4″ × 3″ × ½″ fillet	5.8
Frozen:		
(Banquet)	8¾-oz. dinner	45.4
(Mrs. Paul's) breaded and fried	2-oz. fillet	11.8

Food and Description	Measure or Quantity	Carbohydrates (grams)
(Swanson) fillet almondine	7½-oz. entree	9.0
(Van de Kamp's) batter dipped, french fried	2-oz. piece	8.0
(Weight Watchers) with stuffing, 2-compartment	7-oz. pkg.	14.1
Smoked	4-oz. serving	0.
HALIBUT:		
Broiled	4″ × 3″ × ½″ steak	0.
Frozen (Van de Kamp's) batter dipped, french fried	½ of 8-oz. pkg.	17.0
HAM:		
Canned:		
(Hormel):		
Chunk	6¾-oz. serving	1.5
Chopped	¼ of 12-oz. can	.2
Patties	1 patty	.4
(Oscar Mayer) *Jubilee*, extra lean, cooked	1-oz. serving	.1
(Swift):		
Hostess	3½-oz. slice	.8
Premium	1¾-oz. slice	.3
Deviled:		
(Libby's)	1 oz.	0.
(Underwood)	1 T.	Tr.
Packaged:		
(Eckrich) cooked, sliced	1.2-oz. slice	.7
(Hormel):		
Black or red peppered	.8-oz. slice	.1
Cooked	.8-oz. slice	.1
(Oscar Mayer):		
Chopped	1-oz. slice	.9
Cooked, smoked	¾-oz. slice	0.
Jubilee, steak, boneless, 95% fat free	2-oz. steak	0.
HAMBURGER (*See McDONALD'S, BURGER KING, DAIRY QUEEN, WHITE CASTLE*, etc.)		
HAMBURGER MIX:		
*Hamburger Helper (General Mills):		
Beef noodle	⅕ of pkg.	25.0
Cheeseburger	⅕ of pkg.	28.0
Hash	⅕ of pkg.	24.0
Lasagna	⅕ of pkg.	33.0
Potatoes au gratin	⅕ of pkg.	27.0
Rice oriental	⅕ of pkg.	35.0
Stew	⅕ of pkg.	23.0

Food and Description	Measure or Quantity	Carbohydrates (grams)
Make A Better Burger (Lipton) mildly seasoned or onion	⅓ pkg.	5.0
HAMBURGER SEASONING MIX:		
*(Durkee)	1 cup	7.5
(French's)	1-oz. pkg.	20.0
HAM AND CHEESE:		
(Hormel) loaf	1-oz. serving	.3
(Oscar Mayer) loaf	1-oz. serving	.6
HAM DINNER, frozen:		
(Banquet)	10-oz. dinner	47.7
(Morton)	10-oz. dinner	56.9
(Swanson) *TV Brand*	10¼-oz. dinner	46.0
HAM SALAD, canned (Carnation)	1½-oz. serving	3.1
HAM SALAD SPREAD (Oscar Mayer)	1 oz.	3.0
HAWAIIAN PUNCH:		
Canned:		
Cherry	6 fl. oz.	22.9
Grape	6 fl. oz.	23.4
Orange	6 fl. oz.	24.4
Red	6 fl. oz.	21.3
*Mix, red punch	8 fl. oz.	25.0
HEADCHEESE (Oscar Mayer)	1-oz. serving	0.
HERRING, canned (Vita):		
Cocktail, drained	8-oz. jar	24.8
In cream sauce	8-oz. jar	18.1
Tastee Bits, drained	8-oz. jar	24.7
HERRING, SMOKED, kippered	4-oz. serving	0.
HICKORY NUT, shelled	1-oz. serving	3.6
HO-HO (Hostess)	1-oz. cake	17.0
HOMINY GRITS:		
Dry:		
(Albers)	1½ oz.	33.0
(Aunt Jemima)	3 T.	22.5
(Quaker):		
Regular	3 T.	22.5
Instant:		
Regular	.8-oz. packet	17.7
With imitation bacon or ham	1-oz. packet	21.6
Cooked	1 cup	27.0
HONEY, strained	1 T.	16.5
HONEYCOMB, cereal (Post)	1⅓ cups	25.3
HONEYDEW	2″ × 7″ wedge	7.2

Food and Description	Measure or Quantity	Carbohydrates (grams)
HORSERADISH:		
Raw, pared	1 oz.	5.6
Prepared (Gold's)	1-oz. serving	.4
HOSTESS O'S (Hostess)	2¼-oz. piece	41.5

I

Food and Description	Measure or Quantity	Carbohydrates (grams)
ICE CREAM: (See also FROZEN DESSERT):		
ICE CREAM (listed either by type, such as sandwich or *Whammy*, or by flavor:		
Bar (Good Humor) vanilla, chocolate coated	3-fl.-oz. piece	12.0
Bar (Heath) *Butter Brickle*, chocolate coated	2½-fl.-oz. piece	18.0
Butter pecan:		
(Breyer's)	¼ pt.	15.0
(Good Humor) bulk	4 fl. oz.	14.0
Cherry, black (Good Humor) bulk	4 fl. oz.	14.0
Chocolate:		
(Baskins-Robbins):		
Regular	1 scoop (2½ fl. oz.)	20.4
Fudge	1 scoop (2½ fl. oz.)	21.3
(Good Humor) bulk	4 fl. oz.	15.0
(Swift's) sweet cream	2¼ fl. oz. (½ cup)	15.8
Chocolate chip (Good Humor)	4 fl. oz.	15.0
Chocolate chip cookie (Good Humor)	1 sandwich	64.0
Chocolate eclair, bar (Good Humor)	3-fl. oz. piece	25.0
Coffee (Breyer's)	¼ pt.	15.0
Eskimo Pie, vanilla with chocolate coating	3-fl.-oz. bar	15.0
Eskimo Thin Mint, with chocolate coating	2-fl.-oz. bar	11.0
Fudge royal (Good Humor) bulk	4 fl. oz.	14.0
Peach (Breyer's)	¼ pt.	18.0
Pralines 'n Cream (Baskins-Robbins)	1 scoop (2½ fl. oz.)	23.7
Sandwich (Good Humor)	2½-oz. piece	34.0
Strawberry:		
(Baskins-Robbins)	1 scoop (2½ fl. oz.)	15.6
(Good Humor) bulk	4 fl. oz.	15.0
Strawberry shortcake (Good Humor)	3-fl.-oz. piece	21.0
Toasted almond bar (Good Humor)	3-fl.-oz. piece	21.0

Food and Description	Measure or Quantity	Carbohydrates (grams)
Toffee fudge swirl (Good Humor) bulk	4 fl. oz.	18.0
Vanilla:		
(Baskins-Robbins) regular	1 scoop (2½ oz.)	15.6
(Good Humor) bulk	4 fl. oz.	14.0
(Swift's) sweet cream	½ cup	15.7
Vanilla-chocolate-strawberry (Good Humor) bulk	4 fl. oz.	14.0
Vanilla fudge swirl (Good Humor) bulk	4 fl. oz.	15.0
Whammy (Good Humor):		
Assorted	1.6-oz. piece	9.0
Chip crunch bar	1.6-oz. piece	10.0
ICE CREAM CONE, cone only (Comet):		
Regular	1 piece	4.0
Rolled sugar	1 piece	9.0
ICE CREAM CUP, cup only (Comet)	1 cup	4.0
***ICE CREAM MIX** (Salada)	1 cup	32.0
ICE MILK:		
Hardened	¼ pt.	14.6
Soft-serve	¼ pt.	19.6
(Meadow Gold) vanilla, 4% fat	¼ pt.	18.0
ITALIAN DINNER, frozen (Banquet)	11-oz. dinner	44.6

J

JELLO PUDDING POPS:		
Banana, butterscotch or vanilla	2-oz. pop	15.6
Chocolate or chocolate fudge	2-oz. pop	16.5
JELLY, sweetened (See also individual flavors) (Crosse & Blackwell) all flavors	1 T.	12.8
JERUSALEM ARTICHOKE, pared	4 oz.	18.9
JOHANNISBERG RIESLING:		
(Deinhard)	3 fl. oz.	4.5
(Inglenook)	3 fl. oz	.9

Food and Description	Measure or Quantity	Carbohydrates (grams)

K

KABOOM, cereal (General Mills)	1 cup	23.0
KALE:		
Boiled, leaves only	4 oz.	6.9
Canned (Sunshine) chopped, solids & liq.	½ cup	2.8
Frozen:		
(Birds Eye) chopped	⅓ of pkg.	4.6
(McKenzie) chopped	⅓ of pkg.	5.0
(Southland) chopped	⅕ of 16-oz. pkg.	5.0
KARO SYRUP (See SYRUP)		
KEFIR (Alta-Dena Dairy):		
Plain	1 cup	13.0
Flavored	1 cup	24.0
KIDNEY:		
Beef, braised	4 oz.	.9
Calf, raw	4 oz.	.1
Lamb, raw	4 oz.	1.0
KIELBASA:		
(Eckrich) skinless	2-oz. serving	2.0
(Hormel) Kolbase	2-oz. serving	1.2
(Vienna)	2-oz. serving	1.1
KING VITAMAN, cereal (Quaker)	1¼ cups	23.2
KIRSCH, liqueur (Garnier)	1 fl. oz.	8.8
KIX, cereal	1½ cups	24.0
KNOCKWURST (Best's Kosher; Oscherwitz):		
Regular	3-oz. piece	3.0
Beef	3-oz. piece	2.9
***KOOL-AID** (General Foods):		
Unsweetened	8 fl. oz.	25.0
Pre-Sweetened:		
All flavors except tropical punch	8 fl. oz.	23.2
Tropical punch	8 fl. oz.	24.5
KUMQUAT, flesh & skin	5 oz.	19.4

L

LAMB	any quantity	0.
LASAGNA:		
Canned:		
(Hormel) *Short Orders*	7½-oz. can	24.0

Food and Description	Measure or Quantity	Carbohydrates (grams)
(Nalley's)	8-oz. serving	25.0
Frozen:		
(Green Giant):		
Baked:		
Regular, with meat sauce	12-oz. entree	42.3
Chicken	12-oz. entree	47.0
Boil 'n Bag	9-oz. entree	43.5
(Swanson):		
Regular, with meat in tomato sauce	13¼-oz. entree	45.0
Hungry Man, with meat	17 ¾-oz. dinner	90.0
TV Brand	13-oz. dinner	54.0
(Weight Watchers)	12 ¾-oz. meal	49.3
LEEKS	4 oz.	12.7
LEMON:		
Whole	2 ⅛" lemon	11.7
Peeled	2 ⅛" lemon	6.1
LEMONADE:		
Canned:		
Capri Sun	6 ¾ fl. oz.	23.3
Country Time	6 fl. oz.	17.2
(Hi-C)	6 fl. oz.	17.0
Chilled (Minute Maid) regular or pink	6 fl. oz.	18.0
*Frozen:		
Country Time, regular or pink	6 fl. oz.	18.0
Minute Maid	6 fl. oz.	19.6
*Mix:		
Country Time, regular or pink	6 fl. oz.	16.6
(Hi-C)	6 fl. oz.	19.0
Kool Aid, sweetened, regular or pink	6 fl. oz.	18.8
Lemon Tree (Lipton)	6 fl. oz.	16.5
(Minute Maid) regular or pink	6 fl. oz.	20.0
LEMON JUICE:		
Canned, *ReaLemon*	1 T.	1.1
*Frozen (Minute Maid) unsweetened	1 fl. oz.	2.2
*LEMON-LIMEADE, mix		
(Minute Maid)	6 fl. oz.	20.0
LEMON PEEL, candied	1 oz.	22.9
LEMON-PEPPER SEASONING		
(French's)	1 tsp.	1.0
LENTIL, cooked, drained	½ cup	19.5
LETTUCE:		
Bibb or Boston	4" head	4.1

Food and Description	Measure or Quantity	Carbohydrates (grams)
Cos or Romaine, shredded or broken into pieces	½ cup	.8
Grand Rapids, Salad Bowl or Simpson	2 large leaves	1.8
Iceberg, New York or Great Lakes	¼ of 4 ¾" head	3.3
LIFE, cereal (Quaker) regular or cinnamon	⅔ cup	19.7
LIL' ANGELS (Hostess)	1-oz. piece	14.2
LIME, peeled	2" dia.	4.9
*LIMEADE, frozen (Minute Maid)	6 fl. oz.	20.1
LIME JUICE, *ReaLime*	1 T.	.5
LIVER:		
Beef:		
Fried	6½" × 2⅜" × ⅜" slice	4.5
Cooked (Swift)	3.2-oz. serving	3.1
Calf, fried	6½" × 2⅜" × ⅜" slice	3.4
Chicken, simmered	2" × 2" × ⅝" liver	.8
LIVERWURST SPREAD (Underwood)	1-oz. serving	1.2
LOBSTER:		
Cooked, meat only	1 cup	.4
Canned, meat only	4-oz. serving	.3
Frozen, South African lobster tail:		
3 in 8-oz. pkg.	1 piece	.2
4 in 8-oz. pkg.	1 piece	.1
5 in 8-oz. pkg.	1 piece	<1
LOBSTER NEWBURG	1 cup	12.8
LOBSTER PASTE, canned	1-oz. serving	.4
LOBSTER SALAD	4-oz. serving	2.6
LOG CABIN SYRUP (See SYRUP)		
LONG ISLAND TEA Cocktail, canned (Mr. Boston)	3 fl. oz.	7.5
LOQUAT, fresh, flesh only	2 oz.	7.0
LUCKY CHARMS, cereal (General Mills)	1 cup	24.0
LUNCHEON MEAT (See also individual listings, e.g., BOLOGNA, HAM, etc.)		
All meat (Oscar Mayer)	1-oz. slice	.4
Bar-B-Que loaf (Oscar Mayer) 90% fat free	1-oz. slice	1.4
Beef honey roll sausage (Oscar Mayer) 90% fat free	.8-oz. slice	.7
Beef, jellied (Hormel) loaf	1.2-oz. slice	0.
Ham & cheese (See HAM & CHEESE)		

Food and Description	Measure or Quantity	Carbohydrates (grams)
Ham roll sausage (Oscar Mayer)	.8-oz. slice	.5
Ham roll sausage (Oscar Mayer)	1-oz. slice	.6
Honey loaf:		
(Eckrich)	1-oz. slice	1.8
(Hormel)	1-oz. slice	.6
(Oscar Mayer) 95% fat free	1-oz. slice	1.1
Liver cheese (Oscar Mayer)	1.3-oz. slice	.6
Liver loaf (Hormel)	1-oz. slice	.6
Luxury loaf (Oscar Mayer) 95% fat free	1-oz. slice	1.5
Meat loaf	1-oz. serving	.9
New England brand sliced sausage:		
(Hormel)	1-oz. slice	.2
(Oscar Mayer) 92% fat free	.5-oz. slice	.3
(Oscar Mayer) 92% fat free	.8-oz. slice	.5
Old fashioned loaf:		
(Eckrich)	1-oz. slice	2.0
(Oscar Mayer)	1-oz. slice	2.3
Olive loaf:		
(Hormel)	1-oz. slice	1.5
(Oscar Mayer)	1-oz. slice	2.8
Peppered loaf:		
(Hormel)	1-oz. serving	.4
(Oscar Mayer) 93% fat free	1-oz. slice	1.3
Pickle loaf:		
(Eckrich)	1-oz. slice	1.5
(Hormel)	1-oz. slice	1.3
Pickle & pimiento (Oscar Mayer)	1-oz. slice	3.0
Picnic loaf (Oscar Mayer)	1-oz. slice	1.6
Spiced (Hormel)	1-oz. serving	.5

M

Food and Description	Measure or Quantity	Carbohydrates (grams)
MACADAMIA NUT (Royal Hawaiian)	1 oz.	4.5
MACARONI:		
Cooked:		
8-10 minutes, firm	1 cup	39.1
14-20 minutes, tender	1 cup	32.2
Canned:		
(Franco-American): *Beefy Mac*, & beef	7½-oz. can	30.0
Pizz Os	7½-oz. can	35.0
(Nalley's)	8-oz. serving	29.5

Food and Description	Measure or Quantity	Carbohydrates (grams)
Frozen:		
(Banquet) & beef: regular	12-oz. dinner	55.1
Buffet Supper	2-lb. pkg.	106.4
(Swanson) *TV Brand*, & beef	12-oz. dinner	46.0
MACARONI & CHEESE:		
Canned:		
(Franco-American) regular or elbow	7⅜-oz. serving	24.0
(Hormel) *Short Orders*	7½-oz. can	22.0
Frozen:		
(Banquet):		
Buffet Supper	2-lb. pkg.	110.9
Dinner	12-oz. dinner	45.6
(Green Giant) Boil 'N Bag	9-oz. entree	35.8
(Swanson):		
Regular	12-oz. entree	43.0
TV Brand	12¼-oz. dinner	48.0
Mix:		
(Golden Grain) deluxe	¼ of 7¼-oz. pkg.	38.1
*(Lipton)	¼ of pkg.	25.0
*(Prince)	¾ cup	34.6
MACARONI & CHEESE PIE, frozen (Swanson)	7-oz. pie	25.0
MACARONI SALAD, canned (Nalley's)	4-oz. serving	15.9
MACKEREL, Atlantic, broiled, with fat	8½″ × 2½″ × ½″ fillet	0.
MADEIRA WINE (Leacock)	3 fl. oz.	6.3
MAI TAI COCKTAIL:		
Canned:		
(National Distillers) *Duet* 12½% alcohol	8-fl.-oz. can	28.8
(Party Tyme) 12½% alcohol	2 fl. oz.	5.7
Mix:		
Dry (Bar-Tender's; Holland House)	1 serving	17.0
Liquid, canned (Holland House)	1½ fl. oz.	11.8
MALTED MILK MIX (Carnation):		
Chocolate	3 heaping tsps.	18.0
Natural	3 heaping tsps.	15.8
MALT LIQUOR, *Champale*, regular	12 fl. oz.	12.2
MALT-O-MEAL, cereal	1 T.	7.3
MANDARIN ORANGE (See TANGERINE)		
MANGO, fresh	1 med. mango	22.5

Food and Description	Measure or Quantity	Carbohydrates (grams)
MANGO NECTAR (Libby's)	6 fl. oz.	14.0
MANHATTAN COCKTAIL:		
Canned (Mr. Boston) 20% alcohol	3 fl. oz.	6.3
Mix, dry (Bar-Tender's)	1 serving	5.6
MAPLE SYRUP (See SYRUP, Maple)		
MARGARINE:		
Regular	1 pat (1″ × 1.3″ × 1″, 5 grams)	Tr.
(Mazola)	1 T.	.2
MARGARINE, IMITATION OR DIETETIC (Promise)	1 T.	.1
MARGARINE, WHIPPED (Blue Bonnet; Miracle; Parkay)	1 T.	0.
MARGARITA COCKTAIL:		
Canned (Mr. Boston):		
Regular, 12½% alcohol	3 fl. oz.	10.8
Strawberry, 12½% alcohol	3 fl. oz.	18.9
Mix:		
Dry (Bar-Tender's)	1 serving	17.3
Liquid (Holland House)	1½ fl. oz.	14.2
MARINADE MIX:		
Chicken (Adolph's)	1-oz. packet	14.4
Meat:		
(Durkee)	1-oz. pkg.	9.0
(French's)	1-oz. pkg.	16.0
MARJORAM (French's)	1 tsp.	.8
MARMALADE:		
Sweetened:		
(Keiller)	1 T.	14.9
(Smucker's)	1 T.	13.5
Dietetic:		
(Featherweight)	1 T.	4.0
(Smucker's) imitation	1 T.	6.0
(S&W) *Nutradiet*	1 T.	3.0
MARSHMALLOW FLUFF	1 heaping tsp.	14.4
MARSHMALLOW KRISPIES cereal (Kellogg's)	1¼ cups	33.0
MARTINI COCKTAIL:		
Gin, canned (Mr. Boston) extra dry, 20% alcohol	3 fl. oz.	0.
Gin, mix, liquid (Holland House)	2 fl. oz.	5.1
Vodka, canned (Mr. Boston) 20% alcohol	3 fl. oz.	.9
MASA HARINA (Quaker)	⅓ cup	27.4
MASA TRIGO (Quaker)	⅓ cup	24.7

Food and Description	Measure or Quantity	Carbohydrates (grams)
MATZO (Horowitz Margareten) regular	1 matzo	28.1
MAYONNAISE:		
Real *Hellmann's* (Best Foods)	1 T.	.1
Imitation or dietetic:		
(Diet Delight) *Mayo-Lite*	1 T.	0.
(Featherweight) *Soyamaise*	1 T.	0.
(Tillie Lewis) *Tasti-Diet*,		
Maylonaise	1 T.	1.0
(Weight Watchers)	1 T.	1.0
MAYPO, cereal:		
30-second	¼ cup	16.4
Vermont-style	¼ cup	22.0
McDONALD'S:		
Big Mac	1 hamburger	40.6
Biscuit:		
Ham	1 piece	43.0
Sausage	1 piece	42.5
Cheeseburger	1 hamburger	29.8
Chicken McNuggets	1 serving	15.4
Cookies:		
Chocolate Chip	1 package	44.8
McDonaldland	1 package	48.7
Egg McMuffin	1 serving	31.0
Egg, Scrambled	1 serving	2.5
English Muffin, with butter	1 muffin	29.5
Filet-O-Fish	1 sandwich	37.4
Grapefruit juice	6 fl. oz.	17.9
Hamburger	1 hamburger	29.5
Hot cakes with butter & syrup	1 serving	93.9
McChicken Sandwich	1 sandwich	39.8
McFeast	1 serving	31.3
McRib	1 sandwich	41.0
Orange juice	6 fl. oz.	19.6
Pie:		
Apple	1 pie	29.3
Cherry	1 pie	32.1
Potato:		
Fried	1 regular order	26.1
Hash browns	1 order	14.0
Quarter Pounder	1 hamburger	32.7
Quarter Pounder with cheese	1 hamburger	32.2
Sausage, pork	1 serving	.6
Shake:		
Chocolate	1 serving	65.5
Strawberry	1 serving	62.1
Vanilla	1 serving	59.6

Food and Description	Measure or Quantity	Carbohydrates (grams)
Sundae:		
Caramel	1 sundae	52.5
Hot Fudge	1 sundae	46.2
Strawberry	1 sundae	46.1
MEATBALL DINNER or ENTREE, frozen:		
(Green Giant)	9.9-oz. entree	54.6
(Swanson) *TV Brand*	9¼-oz. entree	21.0
MEATBALL SEASONING MIX:		
*(Durkee) Italian style	1 cup	4.5
(French's)	1½-oz. pkg.	28.0
MEATBALL STEW, canned:		
Dinty Moore	7½-oz. serving	15.1
(Libby's)	12-oz. serving	24.3
(Nalley's)	8-oz. serving	18.2
MEAT LOAF DINNER, frozen:		
(Banquet):		
Regular	11-oz. dinner	29.0
Man-Pleaser	19-oz. dinner	63.6
(Morton) *Country Table*	15-oz. dinner	59.7
(Swanson):		
TV Brand	10 ¾-oz. dinner	48.0
TV Brand, with tomato sauce and whipped potatoes	9-oz. entree	28.0
MEAT LOAF SEASONING MIX (French's)	1½-oz. pkg.	40.0
MEAT, POTTED (Libby's)	1-oz. serving	0.
MEAT SEASONING, dietetic (Featherweight)	¼ tsp.	Tr.
MEAT TENDERIZER (Adolph's)	1 tsp.	.5
MELBA TOAST, salted (Old London):		
Garlic, onion or white rounds	1 piece	1.8
Pumpernickel, rye, wheat or white	1 piece	3.4
Sesame, flat	1 piece	3.5
MELON BALL, in syrup, frozen	½ cup	18.2
MEXICAN DINNER, frozen:		
(Banquet) combination	12-oz. dinner	72.1
(Swanson) *TV Brand*,	16-oz. dinner	66.0
(Van de Kamp's) combination	11-oz. dinner	49.0
MILK, CONDENSED, *Dime Brand; Eagle Brand, Magnolia Brand*	1 T.	10.4
*MILK, DRY, non-fat, instant (Alba; Carnation; Pet)	1 cup	12.0
MILK, EVAPORATED:		

Food and Description	Measure or Quantity	Carbohydrates (grams)
Regular:		
(Carnation)	4 fl. oz.	3.1
(Pet)	1 fl. oz.	3.1
Filled:		
Dairymate	½ cup	12.0
(Pet)	½ cup	12.0
Low fat (Carnation)	1 fl. oz.	3.0
Skimmed:		
(Carnation)	1 fl. oz.	3.5
Pet 99	1 fl. oz.	3.5
MILK, FRESH:		
Buttermilk (Friendship)	8 fl. oz.	12.0
Chocolate (Dairylea)	8 fl. oz.	25.5
Low Fat, *Viva*, 2% fat	8 fl. oz.	12.0
Skim (Dairylea; Meadow Gold)	1 cup	11.0
Whole:		
(Dairylea)	1 cup	11.0
(Meadow Gold)	1 cup	11.0
MILK, GOAT, whole	1 cup	11.2
MILK, HUMAN	1 oz.	2.7
MILNOT, dairy vegetable blend	1 fl. oz.	3.1
MINERAL WATER (Schweppes)	6 fl. oz.	0.
MINI-WHEATS, cereal	1 biscuit	6.0
MINT LEAVES	½ oz.	.8
MOLASSES:		
Barbados	1 T.	13.3
Blackstrap	1 T.	10.4
Dark (Brer Rabbit)	1 T.	10.6
Light	1 T.	12.4
Medium	1 T.	11.4
Unsulphured (Grandma's)	1 T.	15.0
MORTADELLA, sausage	1 oz.	.2
MOSELLE WINE (Great Western)	3 fl. oz.	2.9
MOST, cereal (Kellogg's)	½ cup	22.0
MOUSSE, canned, dietetic (Featherweight) chocolate	½ cup	14.0
MUFFIN:		
Blueberry:		
(Hostess)	1 ¾-oz. muffin	21.9
(Pepperidge Farm)	1.9-oz. muffin	27.0
Bran (Arnold) *Bran'Nola*	2.3-oz. muffin	30.0
Corn:		
(Pepperidge Farm)	1.9-oz. muffin	27.0
(Thomas')	2-oz. muffin	25.8
English:		
(Arnold) extra crisp	2.3-oz. muffin	30.0

Food and Description	Measure or Quantity	Carbohydrates (grams)
(Pepperidge Farm):		
Plain	2-oz. muffin	26.0
Cinnamon apple	2-oz. muffin	27.0
Wheat	2-oz. muffin	25.0
Roman Meal	2⅓-oz. muffin	29.8
(Thomas') regular or frozen	2-oz. muffin	25.7
(Wonder)	2-oz. muffin	26.1
Orange-cranberry (Pepperidge Farm)	21-oz. muffin	30.0
Plain	1.4-oz. muffin	16.9
Raisin (Arnold)	2.5-oz. muffin	35.0
Sourdough (Wonder)	2-oz. muffin	25.6
MUFFIN MIX:		
Blueberry:		
*(Betty Crocker) wild	1 muffin	18.0
(Duncan Hines)	¹⁄₁₂ of pkg.	17.0
Bran (Duncan Hines)	¹⁄₁₂ of pkg.	16.3
Corn:		
*(Betty Crocker)	1 muffin	25.0
*(Dromedary)	1 muffin	20.0
*(Flako)	1 muffin	23.0
MULLIGAN STEW, canned, *Dinty Moore, Short Orders*	7½-oz. can	14.0
MUSCATEL WINE (Gallo) 14% alcohol	3 fl. oz.	7.9
MUSHROOM:		
Raw, whole	½ lb.	9.7
Raw, trimmed, sliced	½ cup	1.5
Canned:		
(Green Giant)	2-oz. serving	1.9
(Shady Oaks)	4-oz. can	2.0
Frozen (Green Giant) whole, in butter sauce	3-oz. serving	3.6
MUSHROOM, CHINESE, dried	1 oz.	18.9
MUSSEL, in shell	1 lb.	7.2
MUSTARD:		
Powder (French's)	1 tsp.	.3
Prepared:		
Brown (French's; Gulden's; *Grey Poupon*)	1 tsp.	.3
Dijon, *Grey Poupon*	1 tsp.	Tr.
Horseradish (Nalley's)	1 tsp.	.3
Yellow (Gulden's)	1 tsp.	.4
MUSTARD GREENS:		
Canned (Sunshine) solids & liq.	½ cup	3.2

Food and Description	Measure or Quantity	Carbohydrates (grams)
Frozen:		
(Birds Eye)	⅓ of pkg.	3.2
(McKenzie)	⅓ of pkg.	3.0
(Seabrook Farms)	⅓ of pkg.	3.4
(Southland)	⅕ of 16-oz. pkg.	3.0
MUSTARD SPINACH:		
Raw	1 lb.	17.7
Boiled, drained, no added salt	4-oz. serving	3.2

N

NATURAL CEREAL:		
Heartland, any flavor	¼ cup	18.0
(Quaker):		
Hot, whole wheat	⅓ cup	21.8
100%	¼ cup	17.4
100% with apple & cinnamon	¼ cup	18.0
NATURE SNACKS (Sun-Maid):		
Carob Crunch	1 oz.	16.8
Raisin Crunch	1 oz.	19.7
Rocky Road	1 oz.	19.1
Tahitian Treat	1 oz.	19.4
Yogurt Crunch	1 oz.	19.7
NECTARINE, flesh only	4 oz.	19.4
NOODLE:		
Dry (Pennsylvania Dutch Brand) broad	1 oz.	20.0
Cooked, 1½″ strips	1 cup	37.3
NOODLES & BEEF:		
Canned (Hormel) *Short Orders*	7½-oz. can	15.0
Frozen (Banquet) *Buffet Supper*	2-lb. pkg.	83.6
NOODLE & CHICKEN:		
Canned, *Dinty Moore, Short Orders*	7½-oz. can	15.0
Frozen (Swanson) *TV Brand*	10½-oz. dinner	53.0
NOODLE, CHOW MEIN:		
(Chun King)	⅙ of 5-oz. can	13.0
(La Choy)	½ cup	16.8
NOODLE MIX:		
(Betty Crocker):		
Fettucine Alfredo or Romanoff	¼ of pkg.	23.0
Stroganoff	¼ of pkg.	26.0
NOODLE RONI, parmesano	⅕ of 6-oz. pkg.	
(Lipton) Egg Noodles & Sauce:		
Beef	¼ of pkg.	26.0

Food and Description	Measure or Quantity	Carbohydrates (grams)
Butter or cheese	¼ of pkg.	24.0
Chicken	¼ of pkg.	25.0
*NOODLE, RAMEN (La Choy) canned:		
Beef or chicken	½ of 3-oz. can	27.6
Oriental	½ of 3-oz. can	27.7
NOODLE, RICE (La Choy)	1 oz.	20.6
NOODLE ROMANOFF, frozen (Stouffer's)	⅓ of pkg.	15.9
NUT, MIXED:		
Dry roasted:		
(Flavor House)	1 oz.	5.4
(Planters)	1 oz.	7.0
Oil roasted:		
(Excel) with peanuts	1 oz.	5.4
(Planters)	1 oz.	6.0
NUTMEG (French's)	1 tsp.	.9
NUT*Os (General Mills)	1 T.	3.0
NUTRI-GRAIN, cereal (Kellogg's):		
Corn	½ cup	24.0
Wheat	⅔ cup	24.0
NUTRIMATO (Mott's)	6 fl. oz.	17.0

O

OAT FLAKES, cereal (Post)	⅔ cup	20.6
OATMEAL:		
Dry:		
Regular:		
(Elam's) Scotch Style	1 oz.	18.2
(H-O) old fashioned	1 T.	2.6
(Quaker) old fashioned	⅓ cup	18.5
Instant:		
(H-O):		
Regular, boxed	1 T.	2.6
Regular, packets	1-oz. packet	17.9
With bran & spice	1½-oz. packet	29.0
With country apple & brown sugar	1.1-oz. packet	22.7
With maple & brown sugar flavor	1½-oz. packet	31.8
(Quaker):		
Regular	1-oz. packet	18.1
Apple & cinnamon	1¼-oz. packet	26.0

Food and Description	Measure or Quantity	Carbohydrates (grams)
Bran & raisin	1½-oz. packet	29.2
Maple & brown sugar	1½-oz. packet	31.9
(3-Minute Brand) *Stir'N Eat*:		
Dutch apple brown sugar	1⅛-oz. packet	23.3
Natural flavor	1-oz. packet	18.0
Quick:		
(Harvest Brand)	⅓ cup	18.5
(H-O)	½ cup	22.2
(Quaker) old fashioned	⅓ cup	18.5
(Ralston Purina)	⅓ cup	18.0
(3-Minute Brand)	⅓ cup	18.5
*Cooked, regular	1 cup	23.3
OIL, SALAD or COOKING	Any quantity	0.
OKRA, frozen:		
(Birds Eye) whole	⅓ of pkg.	5.7
(McKenzie) cut	⅓ of pkg.	6.0
(Seabrook Farms) cut	⅓ of pkg.	6.1
(Southland) cut	⅕ of 16-oz. pkg.	5.0
OLD FASHIONED COCKTAIL:		
Canned (Hiram Walker) 62 proof	3 fl. oz.	3.0
Mix, dry (Bar-Tender's)	1 serving	4.7
OLIVE:		
Green	4 med. or 3 extra large or 2 giant	.2
Ripe, Mission	3 small or 2 large	.3
OMELET, frozen (Swanson) *TV Brand,* Spanish style	7¾-oz. entree	16.0
ONION:		
Raw	2½" onion	8.7
Boiled, pearl onion	½ cup	6.0
Canned (Durkee) *O & C:*		
Boiled	¼ of 16-oz. jar	8.0
Creamed	¼ of 15½-oz. can	65.9
Dehydrated (Gilroy) flakes	1 tsp.	1.3
Frozen:		
(Birds Eye):		
Chopped	1 oz.	2.0
Creamed	⅓ of pkg.	11.4
Whole	⅓ of pkg.	9.6
(Green Giant) cheese sauce	⅓ of pkg.	5.8
(Mrs. Paul's) french-fried rings	½ of 5-oz. pkg.	21.2
(Southland) chopped	⅕ of 10-oz. pkg.	5.0
ONION BOUILLON:		
(Herb-Ox)	1 cube	1.3
MBT	1 packet	2.0
ONION, GREEN	1 small onion	.9

Food and Description	Measure or Quantity	Carbohydrates (grams)
ONION SALAD SEASONING		
(French's) instant	1 T.	3.0
ONION SOUP (See SOUP, Onion)		
***ON*YOS** (General Mills)	1 T.	3.0
ORANGE:		
Peeled	½ cup	15.5
Sections	4 oz.	14.4
ORANGE-APRICOT JUICE		
COCKTAIL, *Musselman's*	8 fl. oz.	23.0
ORANGE DRINK:		
Canned:		
Capri Sun	6 ¾-oz. can	26.1
(Hi-C)	8 fl. oz.	23.0
(Lincoln)	8 fl. oz.	24.0
*Mix (Hi-C)	8 fl. oz.	22.7
ORANGE EXTRACT (Virginia		
Dare)	1 tsp.	0.
ORANGE-GRAPEFRUIT JUICE:		
Canned (Del Monte):		
Sweetened	6 fl. oz.	21.1
Unsweetened	6 fl. oz.	18.3
*Frozen (Minute Maid)		
unsweetened	6 fl. oz.	19.1
ORANGE JUICE:		
Canned:		
(Del Monte) sweetened	6 fl. oz.	17.4
(Libby's) unsweetened	6 fl. oz.	20.0
(Sunkist) unsweetened	½ cup	14.0
(Texsun) sweetened	6 fl. oz.	20.0
Chilled (Minute Maid)	6 fl. oz.	19.7
*Frozen:		
Bright & Early, imitation	6 fl. oz.	21.6
(Minute Maid) unsweetened	6 fl. oz.	20.5
(Snow Crop)	6 fl. oz.	20.5
ORANGE PEEL, candied	1 oz.	22.9
ORANGE-PINEAPPLE DRINK,		
canned (Lincoln)	8 fl. oz.	24.0
ORANGE-PINEAPPLE JUICE,		
canned (Texsun)	6 fl. oz.	21.0
ORANGE-PINEAPPLE JUICE		
COCKTAIL, *Musselman's*	8 fl. oz.	23.0
***ORANGE PLUS** (Birds Eye)	6 fl. oz.	23.6
ORANGE SPREAD, dietetic (Estee)	1 tsp.	1.9
OVALTINE, chocolate or malt	¾ oz.	17.9
OVEN FRY (General Foods):		
Crispy crumb for pork	4.2-oz. envelope	78.0

Food and Description	Measure or Quantity	Carbohydrates (grams)
Extra crispy for chicken	4.2-oz. envelope	76.5
Traditional pork	5.3-oz. envelope	98.9
OYSTER:		
Raw:		
Eastern	19-31 small or 13-19 med.	8.2
Pacific & Western	6-9 small or 4-6 med.	15.4
Canned (Bumble) shelled, whole, solids & liq.	1 cup	15.4
Fried	4 oz.	21.1
OYSTER STEW, home recipe	½ cup	5.6

P

Food and Description	Measure or Quantity	Carbohydrates (grams)
PAC-MAN CEREAL (General Mills)	1 cup	25.0
***PANCAKE BATTER, FROZEN**		
(Aunt Jemima):		
Plain or buttermilk	4" pancake	14.1
Blueberry	4" pancake	13.8
PANCAKE & SAUSAGE, frozen (Swanson)	6-oz. entree	48.0
***PANCAKE & WAFFLE MIX:**		
Plain:		
(Aunt Jemima):		
Complete	4" pancake	15.7
Original	4" pancake	8.7
(Log Cabin):		
Complete	4" pancake	11.2
Original	4" pancake	8.7
(Pillsbury) *Hungry Jack:*		
Complete, bulk or packets	4" pancake	12.3
Extra Lights	4" pancake	9.3
Panshakes	4" pancake	14.3
Blueberry (Pillsbury) *Hungry Jack*	4" pancake	13.3
Buckwheat (Aunt Jemima)	4" pancake	8.3
Buttermilk:		
(Aunt Jemima):		
Regular	4" pancake	13.3
Complete	4" pancake	15.3
(Betty Crocker):		
Regular	4" pancake	13.0
Complete	4" pancake	13.7
(Pillsbury) *Hungry Jack*, complete	4" pancake	12.0

Food and Description	Measure or Quantity	Carbohydrates (grams)
Whole wheat (Aunt Jemima)	4" pancake	10.7
Dietetic:		
(Featherweight)	4" pancake	8.0
(Tillie Lewis) *Tasti-Diet*	4" pancake	8.7
PANCAKE & WAFFLE SYRUP (See SYRUP, Pancake & Waffle)		
PAPAYA, fresh:		
Cubed	½ cup	9.1
Juice	4 oz.	18.8
PAPRIKA (French's)	1 tsp.	1.1
PARSLEY:		
Fresh, chopped	1 T.	.3
Dried (French's)	1 tsp.	.6
PASSION FRUIT, giant, whole	1 lb.	11.3
PASTINA, egg	1 oz.	20.4
PASTRAMI:		
(Eckrich) sliced	1-oz. serving	1.3
(Vienna)	1-oz. serving	0.
PASTRY SHEET, PUFF, frozen (Pepperidge Farm)	4.3-oz. sheet	45.0
PASTRY SHELL, frozen (Pepperidge Farm)	1 patty shell	17.0
PÂTÉ:		
De foie gras	1 T.	.7
Liver (Hormel)	1 T.	.3
PDQ:		
Chocolate	1 T.	15.1
Strawberry	1 T.	15.0
PEA, green:		
Boiled	½ cup	9.9
Canned, regular pack, solids & liq.:		
(Del Monte):		
Early	½ cup	9.9
Seasoned	½ cup	9.8
(Green Giant):		
Early, with onions	½ cup	10.4
Sweet	½ cup	11.1
(Libby's) sweet	½ cup	11.6
(Stokely-Van Camp) early	½ cup	12.5
Canned, dietetec pack, solids & liq.:		
(Diet Delight)	½ cup	8.0
(Featherweight) sweet	½ cup	12.0
(S&W) *Nutradiet*, sweet	½ cup	8.0
Frozen:		
(Birds Eye):		
Regular	⅓ of pkg.	13.3

Food and Description	Measure or Quantity	Carbohydrates (grams)
In cream sauce	⅓ of pkg.	14.3
With sliced mushrooms	⅓ of pkg.	12.9
(Green Giant):		
Creamed	3.3 oz.	10.4
Early & sweet in butter sauce	3.3 oz.	11.1
Sweet, *Harvest Fresh*	4 oz.	15.1
(McKenzie) regular	⅓ of pkg.	13.0
(Seabrook Farms)	⅓ of pkg.	13.1
PEA & CARROT:		
Canned, regular pack, solids & liq.:		
(Del Monte)	½ cup	9.4
(Libby's)	½ cup	10.3
Canned, dietetic pack, solids & liq.:		
(Diet Delight)	½ cup	6.0
(S&W) *Nutradiet*	½ cup	7.0
Frozen (Birds Eye)	⅓ of pkg.	11.2
PEA, CROWDER, frozen		
(Southland)	⅕ of 16-oz. pkg.	21.0
PEA POD:		
Boiled, drained solids	4 oz.	10.8
Frozen (La Choy)	6-oz. pkg.	20.4
PEA SOUP (See SOUP, Pea)		
PEACH:		
Fresh, with thin skin	2" peach	9.6
Fresh, slices	½ cup	8.2
Canned, regular pack, solids & liq.:		
(Del Monte):		
Cling	½ cup	22.8
Spiced	7¼ oz.	41.2
(Libby's):		
Halves, heavy syrup	½ cup	25.4
Sliced, heavy syrup	½ cup	24.7
Canned, dietetic pack, solids & liq.:		
(Del Monte) *Lite*, Cling	½ cup	12.6
(Diet Delight), cling, syrup pack	½ cup	14.0
(Featherweight):		
Cling or Freestone, juice pack	½ cup	12.0
Cling, water pack	½ cup	8.0
(Libby's) water pack, Lite	½ cup	13.0
(S&W) *Nutradiet:*		
Cling, juice pack	½ cup	14.0
Cling, water pack	½ cup	8.0
Freestone, juice pack	½ cup	14.0
Frozen (Birds Eye) sliced	5 oz.	34.0
PEACH BUTTER (Smucker's)	1 T.	16.0

Food and Description	Measure or Quantity	Carbohydrates (grams)
PEACH DRINK (Hi-C):		
Canned	6 fl. oz.	23.0
*Mix	6 fl. oz.	18.0
PEACH LIQUEUR (DeKuyper)	1 fl. oz.	8.3
PEACH NECTAR (Libby's)	6 fl. oz.	23.0
PEACH PRESERVE OR JAM:		
Sweetened (Smucker's)	1 T.	13.5
Dietetic:		
(Featherweight)	1 T.	4.0
(Featherweight) artificially sweetened	1 T.	1.0
PEACH SPREAD, dietetic (Tillie Lewis) *Tasti-Diet*	1 T.	3.0
PEANUT:		
Dry roasted:		
(Fisher)	1 oz.	5.0
(Frito-Lay)	1 oz.	6.2
(Planters)	1 oz.	6.0
Oil roasted (Planters)	1 oz. (jar)	5.0
PEANUT BUTTER:		
Regular:		
(Elam's) Natural with defatted wheat germ	1 T.	2.1
(Jif) creamy	1 T.	2.7
(Peter Pan):		
Crunchy	1 T.	3.0
Smooth	1 T.	3.1
(Planters) crunchy or smooth	1 T.	3.0
(Skippy):		
Creamy	1 T.	3.0
Super chunk	1 T.	2.9
(Smucker's) creamy, crunchy or natural	1 T.	3.0
Dietetic:		
(Featherweight) low sodium	1 T.	2.0
(Peter Pan) low sodium	1 T.	2.3
(S&W) *Nutradiet*, low sodium	1 T.	2.0
PEANUT BUTTER BAKING CHIPS (Reese's)	3 T. (1 oz.)	12.8
PEAR:		
Whole	3″ × 2½″ pear	25.4
Canned, regular pack, solids & liq.:		
(Del Monte)	½ cup	21.3
(Libby's)	½ cup	22.7
Canned, dietetic pack, solids & liq.:		
(Del Monte) *Lite*	½ cup	13.9

Food and Description	Measure or Quantity	Carbohydrates (grams)
(Featherweight):		
Bartlett, juice pack	½ cup	16.0
Bartlett, water pack	½ cup	10.0
(Libby's) water pack	½ cup	15.0
(S&W) *Nutradiet:*		
Juice pack	½ cup	15.0
Water pack	½ cup	10.0
Dried (Sun-Maid)	½ cup	70.0
PEAR NECTAR (Libby's)	6 fl. oz.	11.5
PEAR-PASSION FRUIT NECTAR		
(Libby's)	6 fl. oz.	14.0
PEBBLES, cereal:		
Cocoa	⅞ cup	24.4
Fruity	⅞ cup	24.5
PECAN:		
Halves	6–7 pieces	1.0
Roasted, dry:		
(Fisher) salted	1 oz.	4.5
(Planters)	1 oz.	5.0
PECTIN, FRUIT:		
Certo	6-oz.	4.8
Sure-Jell	1 ¾ oz.	42.5
PEP, cereal (Kellogg's)	¾ cup	23.0
PEPPER:		
Black (French's)	1 tsp.	1.5
Lemon (Durkee)	1 tsp.	.2
Seasoned (French's)	1 tsp.	1.0
PEPPER, CHILI, canned:		
(Del Monte):		
Green, whole	½ cup	5.0
Jalapeno or chili, whole	½ cup	6.0
Old El Paso, green, chopped or		
whole	1 oz.	1.4
(Ortega):		
Diced, strips or whole	1 oz.	1.1
Jalapeno, diced or whole	1 oz.	1.7
PEPPERONI:		
(Hormel) sliced	1-oz. serving	.3
(Swift)	1-oz. serving	1.0
PEPPER & ONION, frozen		
(Southland):		
Diced	2 oz.	3.0
Red & green	2 oz.	4.0
PEPPER STEAK, frozen:		
*(Chun King) stir fry	⅓ of pkg.	3.0
(Stouffer's)	5¼-oz. serving	34.9

Food and Description	Measure or Quantity	Carbohydrates (grams)
PEPPER, STUFFED:		
Home recipe	2 ¾" × 2½" pepper with 1⅛ cups stuffing	31.1
Frozen:		
(Green Giant) green, baked	7 oz.	17.1
(Weight Watchers) with veal stuffing	11¾ oz.	22.0
PEPPER, SWEET:		
Raw:		
Green:		
Whole	1 lb.	17.9
Without stem & seeds	1 med. pepper (2.6 oz.)	2.9
Red:		
Whole	1 lb.	25.8
Without stem & seeds	1 med. pepper (2.2 oz.)	2.4
Boiled, green, without salt, drained	1 med. pepper (2.6 oz.)	2.8
Frozen:		
(McKenzie) green	1 oz.	1.0
(Southland):		
Green	2 oz.	3.0
Red & Green	2 oz.	3.0
PERCH, OCEAN:		
Atlantic, raw:		
Whole	1 lb.	0.
Meat only	4 oz.	0.
Pacific, raw, whole	1 lb.	0.
Frozen:		
(Banquet)	8 ¾-oz. dinner	49.8
(Mrs. Paul's) fillet, breaded & fried	2-oz. piece	8.8
(Van de Kamp's)	2-oz. piece	10.0
(Weight Watchers)	6 ½-oz. meal	11.0
PERNOD (Julius Wile)	1 fl. oz.	1.1
PERSIMMON:		
Japanese or Kaki, fresh:		
With seeds	4.4-oz. piece	20.1
Seedless	4.4-oz. piece	20.7
Native, fresh, flesh only	4 oz.	38.0
PHEASANT, raw, meat only	4 oz.	0.
PICKLE:		
Cucumber, fresh or bread & butter:		
(Fannings)	1.2 oz.	3.9

Food and Description	Measure or Quantity	Carbohydrates (grams)
(Featherweight)	1 oz.	3.0
(Nalley's) chips	1 oz.	6.5
Dill:		
(Featherweight) whole, low sodium	1 oz.	1.0
(Nalley's) regular & Polish style	1 oz.	.6
(Smucker's):		
Hamburger sliced	1 slice	0.
Polish, whole	3½" pickle	1.0
Spears	3½" spear	1.0
Hamburger (Nalley's) chips	1 oz.	.6
Kosher dill:		
(Claussen) halves or whole	2 oz.	1.3
(Featherweight) low sodium	1 oz.	1.0
(Nalley's)	2 oz.	1.7
(Smucker's):		
Baby	2 ¾" long pickle	.5
Slices	1 slice	0.
Whole	2½" long pickle	1.0
Sweet:		
(Nalley's):		
Regular	1 oz.	10.5
Nubbins	1 oz.	7.9
(Smucker's):		
Candied mix	1 piece	3.3
Gherkins	2" long pickle	3.5
Whole	2½" long pickle	4.0
Sweet & sour (Claussen) slices	1 slice	.8
PIE:		
Regular:		
Apple:		
Home recipe, two-crust	⅙ of 9" pie	60.2
(Hostess)	4½-oz. pie	51.1
Banana, home recipe, cream or custard	⅙ of 9" pie	46.7
Berry (Hostess)	4½-oz. pie	51.1
Blackberry, home recipe, two-crust	⅙ of 9" pie	54.4
Blueberry:		
Home recipe, two-crust	⅙ of 9" pie	55.1
(Hostess)	4½-oz. pie	49.9
Boston cream, home recipe	1/12 of 8" pie	34.4
Butterscotch, home recipe, one-crust	⅙ of 9" pie	58.2
Cherry:		
Home recipe, two-crust	⅙ of 9" pie	60.7
(Hostess)	4½-oz. pie	56.2

Food and Description	*Measure or Quantity*	*Carbohydrates (grams)*
Chocolate chiffon, home recipe	1/6 of 9" pie	61.2
Chocolate meringue, home recipe	1/6 of 9" pie	46.9
Coconut custard, home recipe	1/6 of 9" pie	37.8
Lemon (Hostess)	4½-oz. pie	52.4
Mince, home recipe, two-crust	1/6 of 9" pie	65.1
Peach (Hostess)	4½-oz. pie	52.4
Pecan (Frito-Lay)	3-oz. serving	53.5
Pumpkin, home recipe, one-crust	1/6 of 9" pie	37.2
Raisin, home recipe, two-crust	1/6 of 9" pie	67.9
Rhubarb, home recipe, two-crust	1/6 of 9" pie	60.4
Strawberry (Hostess)	4½-oz. pie	56.2
Frozen:		
Apple:		
(Banquet)	1/5 of 20-oz. pie	42.6
(Morton):		
Regular	1/6 of 24-oz. pie	40.9
Great Little Desserts	8-oz. pie	88.6
(Sara Lee):		
Regular	1/6 of 31-oz. pie	43.2
Dutch	1/6 of 30-oz. pie	50.6
Banana cream:		
(Banquet)	1/6 of 14-oz. pie	19.9
(Morton):		
Regular	1/6 of 16-oz. pie	19.7
Great Little Desserts	3½-oz. pie	25.8
Blueberry:		
(Banquet)	1/6 of 20-oz. pie	37.5
(Morton):		
Regular	1/6 of 24-oz. pie	38.6
Great Little Desserts	8-oz. pie	86.4
(Sara Lee)	1/6 of 31-oz. pie	44.8
Cherry:		
(Banquet)	1/6 of 20-oz. pie	33.8
(Morton):		
Regular	1/6 of 24-oz. pie	42.0
Great Little Desserts	8-oz. pie	86.4
(Sara Lee)	1/6 of 31-oz. pie	48.0
Chocolate cream:		
(Banquet)	1/6 of 14-oz. pie	21.8
(Morton) regular	1/6 of 16-oz. pie	22.8
Coconut cream:		
(Banquet)	1/6 of 14-oz. pie	19.1
(Morton):		
Regular	1/6 of 16-oz. pie	22.0
Great Little Desserts	2½-oz. pie	28.8

Food and Description	Measure or Quantity	Carbohydrates (grams)
Coconut custard:		
(Banquet)	⅙ of 20-oz. pie	28.2
(Morton) *Great Little Desserts*	6½-oz. pie	53.2
Custard (Banquet)	⅕ of 20-oz. pie	38.2
Lemon cream:		
(Banquet)	⅙ of 14-oz. pie	21.8
(Morton):		
Regular	⅙ of 16-oz. pie	22.0
Great Little Desserts	3½-oz. pie	27.8
Mince:		
(Banquet)	⅙ of 20-oz. pie	38.5
(Morton)	⅙ of 24-oz. pie	45.5
Neapolitan (Morton)	⅙ of 16-oz. pie	23.0
Peach:		
(Banquet)	⅕ of 20-oz. pie	35.9
(Morton)	⅙ of 24-oz. pie	38.7
(Sara Lee)	⅙ of 31-oz. pie	56.2
Pumpkin:		
(Banquet)	⅙ of 20-oz. pie	32.3
(Morton)	⅙ of 24-oz. pie	36.4
(Sara Lee)	⅛ of 45-oz. pie	49.4
Strawberry cream:		
(Banquet)	⅙ of 14-oz. pie	22.5
(Morton)	⅙ of 16-oz. pie	22.0
PIECRUST:		
Home recipe, 9″ pie	1 crust	78.8
Frozen (Banquet) 9″ pie shell:		
Regular	1 crust	61.9
Deep dish	1 crust	78.8
*PIECRUST MIX:		
(Betty Crocker) regular or stick:		
Regular	1⁄16 pkg.	10.0
Stick	⅛ stick	10.0
(Flako)	⅙ of 9″ pie shell	25.2
(Pillsbury) mix or stick	⅙ of 2-crust shell	25.0
PIE FILLING (See also PUDDING OR PIE FILLING):		
Apple (Comstock)	⅙ of 21-oz. can	24.0
Apple rings or slices (See APPLE, canned)		
Apricot (Comstock)	⅙ of 21-oz. can	24.0
Banana cream (Comstock)	⅙ of 21-oz. can	22.0
Blueberry (Comstock)	⅙ of 21-oz. can	26.0
Cherry (Comstock)	⅙ of 21-oz. can	26.0
Coconut cream (Comstock)	⅙ of 21-oz. can	24.0

Food and Description	Measure or Quantity	Carbohydrates (grams)
Coconut custard, home recipe, made with egg yolk & milk	5 oz. (inc. crust)	41.3
Lemon (Comstock)	⅙ of 21-oz. can	33.0
Mincemeat (Comstock)	⅙ of 21-oz. can	36.0
Peach (Comstock)	⅙ of 21-oz. can	27.0
Pineapple (Comstock)	⅙ of 21-oz. can	25.0
Pumpkin (Libby's) (See also PUMPKIN, canned)	1 cup	51.0
Raisin Comstock)	⅙ of 21-oz. can	30.0
Strawberry (Comstock)	⅙ of 21-oz. can	28.0
*PIE MIX (Betty Crocker) Boston cream	⅛ of pie	48.0
PIEROGIES, frozen (Mrs. Paul's):		
Cabbage	5-oz. serving	64.0
Potato & cheese	5-oz. serving	56.6
Sauerkraut, Polish-style	5-oz. serving	60.2
PIGS FEET, pickled	4 oz.	0.
PIMIENTO, canned:		
(Dromedary)	1-oz. serving	2.0
(Ortega)	¼ cup	1.3
(Sunshine) diced or sliced	1 T.	.9
PINA COLADA:		
Canned (Mr. Boston) 12½% alcohol	3 fl. oz.	34.2
Mix:		
Dry (Party Tyme)	½-oz. pkg.	13.2
Liquid (Holland House)	2 fl. oz.	30.0
PINEAPPLE:		
Fresh, slices	½ cup	10.7
Canned, regular pack, solids & liq.:		
(Del Monte) slices, medium	½ cup	22.2
(Dole):		
Chunk, crushed or sliced, juice pack	½ cup	17.5
Chunk, crushed or sliced, heavy syrup	½ cup	24.8
Canned, unsweetened or dietetic, solids & liq.:		
(Del Monte):		
Chunks, juice pack	½ cup	16.8
Crushed, juice pack	½ cup	18.5
Slices, juice pack	½ cup	19.6
(Diet Delight) juice pack	½ cup	18.0
(Featherweight):		
Juice pack	½ cup	18.0
Water pack	½ cup	15.0
(Libby's)	½ cup	16.0

Food and Description	Measure or Quantity	Carbohydrates (grams)
(S&W) *Nutradiet*, slices	1 slice	7.5
PINEAPPLE, CANDIED	1 oz.	22.7
PINEAPPLE & GRAPEFRUIT JUICE DRINK, canned:		
(Del Monte) regular or pink	6 fl. oz.	23.6
(Dole) pink	6 fl. oz.	25.4
(Texsun)	6 fl. oz.	22.0
PINEAPPLE JUICE:		
Canned:		
(Del Monte) with vitamin C	6 fl. oz.	26.3
(Dole)	6 fl. oz.	25.4
(Texsun)	6 fl. oz.	24.0
*Frozen (Minute Maid)	6 fl. oz.	22.7
PINEAPPLE-ORANGE DRINK, canned (Hi-C)	6 fl. oz.	23.0
PINEAPPLE-ORANGE JUICE:		
Canned (Del Monte)	6 fl. oz.	23.8
*Frozen (Minute Maid)	6 fl. oz.	23.0
PINEAPPLE PRESERVE OR JAM, sweetened (Smucker's)	1 T.	13.5
PINE NUT, pignolias, shelled	1 oz.	3.3
PINOT CHARDONNAY WINE (Paul Masson) 12% alcohol	3 fl. oz.	2.4
PISTACHIO NUT:		
In shell	½ cup	6.3
Shelled	¼ cup	5.9
(Fisher) shelled, roasted, salted	1 oz.	5.4
PIZZA PIE:		
Regular, non-frozen:		
Home recipe with cheese	⅛ of 14″ pie	21.2
(Pizza Hut):		
Cheese	½ of 10″ pie	53.2
Pepperoni	½ of 10″ pie	54.4
Pork	½ of 10″ pie	54.4
Frozen:		
Canadian style bacon (Celeste)	8-oz. pie	50.4
Cheese:		
(Celeste)	½ of 7-oz. pie	28.6
(Celeste)	¼ of 19-oz. pie	31.6
(Stouffer's) French bread	½ of 10¼-oz. pkg.	46.0
Totino's	½ of pie	53.0
(Weight Watchers)	6-oz. pie	31.0
Combination:		
(Celeste) Chicago style	¼ of 24-oz. pie	36.2
(La Pizzeria)	½ of 13½-oz. pie	43.0
(Van de Kamp's) thick crust	¼ of 23.4-oz. pie	24.0

Food and Description	Measure or Quantity	Carbohydrates (grams)
(Weight Watchers) deluxe	7¼-oz. pie	27.9
Deluxe:		
(Celeste)	½ of 9-oz. pie	31.3
(Celeste)	¼ of 23½-oz. pie	37.4
(Stouffer's) French bread	½ of 12 ⅜-oz. pkg.	46.0
Hamburger (Stouffer's) French bread	½ of 12¼-oz. pkg.	38.0
Mexican style (Van de Kamp's)	½ of 11-oz. pie	27.0
Pepperoni:		
(Celeste)	½ of 7¼-oz. pie	27.0
(Celeste)	¼ of 20-oz. pie	34.8
(Stouffer's) French bread	½ of 11¼-oz. pkg.	43.8
Totino's	½ of pie	52.0
(Van de Kamp's) thick crust	¼ of 22-oz. pie	38.0
Sausage:		
(Celeste)	½ of 8-oz. pie	29.8
(Celeste)	¼ of 22-oz. pie	34.7
(Stouffer's) French bread	½ of 12-oz. pkg.	44.0
Totino's	½ of pie	54.0
(Weight Watchers)	6¾-oz. pie	29.1
Sausage & mushroom:		
(Celeste)	½ of 9-oz. pie	28.4
(Celeste)	¼ of 24-oz. pie	34.1
(Stouffer's) French bread	½ of 12½-oz. pkg.	40.0
Sicilian style (Celeste) deluxe	¼ of 26-oz. pie	45.4
Suprema (Celeste):		
Regular	½ of 10-oz. pie	26.1
Without meat	½ of 8-oz. pie	24.6
Vegetable (Weight Watchers)	7¼-oz. pie	35.0
PIZZA PIE MIX:		
Regular (Jeno's)	½ of pkg.	67.0
Cheese:		
(Jeno's)	½ of pkg.	62.0
*(Ragu) Pizza Quick	⅛ of 12″ pie	19.0
Skillet Pizza (General Mills)	¼ pkg.	30.0
Pepperoni:		
(Jeno's)	½ of pkg.	67.0
Skillet Pizza (General Mills)	¼ of pkg.	31.0
Sausage, *Skillet Pizza* (General Mills	¼ of pkg.	29.0
PIZZA SAUCE:		
(Contadina):		
Regular	½ cup	10.0
With cheese	½ cup	11.0

Food and Description	Measure or Quantity	Carbohydrates (grams)
(Ragu):		
Regular	5 oz.	15.0
Pizza Quick	5 oz.	13.0
PIZZA SEASONING SPICE		
(French's)	1 tsp.	1.0
PLUM:		
Fresh, Japanese & hybrid	2″ plum	6.9
Fresh, prune-type, halves	½ cup	15.8
Canned, regular pack (Stokely-Van Camp)	½ cup	30.0
Canned, purple, unsweetened or dietetic, solids & liq.:		
(Diet Delight) juice pack	½ cup	19.0
(Featherweight):		
Juice pack	½ cup	18.0
Water pack	½ cup	9.0
(S&W) *Nutradiet*, juice pack	½ cup	20.0
PLUM JELLY (Featherweight)	1 T.	4.0
PLUM PRESERVE OR JAM, sweetened (Smucker's)	1 T.	13.5
P.M. FRUIT DRINK (Mott's)	6 fl. oz.	22.0
POLYNESIAN-STYLE DINNER, frozen (Swanson) *TV Brand*	12-oz. dinner	46.0
POMEGRANATE, whole	1 lb.	41.7
PONDEROSA RESTAURANT:		
A-1 sauce	1 tsp.	1.0
Beef, chopped (patty only)	any size	0.
Beverages:		
Coca-Cola	8 fl. oz.	24.0
Coffee	6 fl. oz.	.5
Dr. Pepper	8 fl. oz.	24.8
Milk:		
Regular	8 fl. oz.	12.0
Chocolate	8 fl. oz.	25.9
Orange drink	8 fl. oz.	30.0
Root beer	8 fl. oz.	25.6
Sprite	8 fl. oz.	24.0
Tab	8 fl. oz.	.1
Tea	6 fl. oz.	.5
Bun:		
Regular	2.4-oz. bun	35.0
Hot dog	1 bun	18.9
Junior	1.4-oz. bun	21.0
Steakhouse Deluxe	2.4-oz. bun	35.0
Butter	1 pat (1 tsp.)	Tr.
Catsup	1 T.	4.3

Food and Description	Measure or Quantity	Carbohydrates (grams)
Chicken strips:		
Adult	2 ¾ oz.	15.8
Child	1.4-oz.	7.9
Cocktail sauce	1½ oz.	14.5
Filet Mignon	3.8 oz. (edible portion)	.2
Filet of Sole, fish only (See also Bun)	3-oz. piece	4.4
Fish, baked	4.9 oz. serving	11.6
Gelatin dessert	½ cup	23.5
Gravy, Au Jus	1 oz.	Tr.
Ham & cheese:		
Bun (See Bun)		
Cheese, Swiss	2 slices (.8 oz.)	.5
Ham	2½ oz.	1.4
Hot dog, child's, meat only (See also Bun)	1.6-oz. hot dog	2.0
Lemon wedge		2.7
Lettuce (See Salad bar)		
Margarine:		
Pat	1 tsp.	Tr.
On potato, as served	½ oz.	.1
Mayonnaise	1 T.	.3
Mustard	1 T.	.9
Mustard sauce, sweet & sour	1 oz.	9.5
New York strip steak	6.1 oz. (edible portion)	0.
Onion, chopped	1 T. (.4 oz.)	.9
Pickle, dill	3 slices (.7 oz.)	.2
Potato:		
Baked	7.2 oz.	32.8
French fries	3 oz.	30.2
Prime Rib	Any size	0.
Pudding:		
Butterscotch	4½ oz.	27.4
Chocolate	4½ oz.	27.1
Vanilla	4½ oz.	27.5
Ribeye	3.2 oz. (edible portion)	0.
Ribeye & Shrimp:		
Ribeye	3.2 oz.	0.
Shrimp	2.2 oz.	6.2
Roll, kaiser	2.2-oz. roll	33.0
Salad bar:		
Bean sprouts	1 oz.	1.4
Beets	1 oz.	.9

Food and Description	Measure or Quantity	Carbohydrates (grams)
Broccoli	1 oz.	1.7
Cabbage, red	1 oz.	2.0
Carrots	1 oz.	2.8
Cauliflower	1 oz.	1.5
Celery	1 oz.	1.1
Chickpeas (Garbanzos)	1 oz.	17.3
Cucumber	1 oz.	1.0
Lettuce	1 oz.	.7
Mushrooms	1 oz.	1.2
Onions, white	1 oz.	2.6
Pepper, green	1 oz.	1.4
Radish	1 oz.	1.0
Tomato	1 oz.	1.3
Salad dressing:		
Blue cheese	1 oz.	2.1
Italian, creamy	1 oz.	2.8
Low calorie	1 oz.	.8
Oil & vinegar	1 oz.	.9
Sweet'n tart	1 oz.	9.2
Thousand island	1 oz.	6.7
Shrimp dinner	7 pieces (3½ oz.)	9.8
Sirloin	any size	0.
Steak sauce	1 oz.	4.6
Tartar sauce	1½ oz.	4.5
T-Bone	4.3 oz. (edible portion)	0.
Tomato (See also Salad bar):		
Slices	2 slices (.9 oz.)	1.2
Whole, small	3.5 oz.	4.7
Topping, whipped	¼ oz.	1.2
Worcestershire sauce	1 tsp.	.9
POPCORN:		
*Home made, popped: (Jiffy Pop)	½ of 5-oz. pkg.	29.8
(Pillsbury) Microwave Popcorn:		
Regular	1 cup	6.5
Butter flavor	1 cup	6.0
Packaged:		
Caramel-coated (Bachman)	1-oz. serving	25.0
Cheese flavored (Bachman)	1-oz. serving	14.0
Cracker Jack	¾-oz. serving	16.7
POP TARTS (*See* TOASTER CAKE OR PASTRY)		
PORK	any quantity	0.
PORK DINNER (Swanson) *TV Brand*	11¼-oz. dinner	20.0
PORK RINDS, *Baken-Ets*	1-oz. serving	1.0

Food and Description	Measure or Quantity	Carbohydrates (grams)
PORK STEAK, BREADED, frozen (Hormel)	3-oz. serving	11.0
PORK, SWEET & SOUR, frozen (La Choy)	½ of 15-oz. pkg.	45.2
PORT WINE:		
(Gallo)	3 fl. oz.	7.8
(Great Western)	3 fl. oz.	11.5
(Louis M. Martini)	6 fl. oz.	2.0
***POSTUM**, instant	6 fl. oz.	2.6
POTATO:		
Cooked:		
Au gratin	½ cup	17.9
Baked, peeled	2½" dia. potato	20.9
Boiled, peeled	4.2-oz. potato	17.7
French-fried	10 pieces	20.5
Hash-browned, home recipe	½ cup	28.4
Mashed, milk & butter added	½ cup	12.1
Canned:		
(Del Monte) drained	1 cup	28.4
(Sunshine) whole, solids & liq.	1 cup	21.0
Frozen:		
(Birds Eye):		
Cottage Fries	2.8-oz. serving	17.3
Crinkle cuts, regular	3-oz. serving	18.4
French fries, regular	3-oz. serving	16.8
Hash browns, shredded	¼ of 12-oz. pkg.	13.1
Tasti Puffs	¼ of 10-oz. pkg.	19.4
Tiny Taters	⅕ of 16-oz. pkg.	22.0
Triangles	1½-oz. serving	5.9
(Green Giant):		
Sliced in butter sauce	3.3 oz.	4.0
& sweet peas in bacon cream sauce	3.3 oz.	12.8
(McKenzie) whole, white	3.2 oz.	13.0
(Seabrook Farms) whole, boiled	3½-oz. serving	14.9
(Southland) whole	4-oz. serving	16.0
(Stouffer's):		
Au gratin	⅓ of pkg.	12.9
Scalloped	⅓ of pkg.	13.9
POTATO & BACON, canned (Hormel) *Short Orders*, au gratin	7½-oz. can	20.0
POTATO & BEEF, canned, *Dinty Moore, Short Orders*, hashed	1½-oz. can	25.0
POTATO CHIP:		
(Bachman) regular, BBQ or sour cream	1 oz.	14.0

Food and Description	Measure or Quantity	Carbohydrates (grams)
(Featherweight) unsalted	1 oz.	14.0
(Frito-Lay's) natural	1 oz.	15.1
Lay's, sour cream & onion flavor	1 oz.	14.0
(Planter's) stackable	1 oz.	17.0
Pringles:		
Regular	1 oz.	11.9
Light	1 oz.	16.8
POTATO & HAM, canned (Hormel)		
Short Orders, scalloped	7½-oz. can	18.0
***POTATO MIX:**		
Au gratin:		
(Betty Crocker)	½ cup	21.0
(French's) *Big Tate,* tangy	½ cup	25.0
(Libby's) *Potato Classics*	¾ cup	22.0
Creamed (Betty Crocker)	½ cup	20.0
Hash browns (Betty Crocker) with onion	½ cup	23.0
Julienne (Betty Crocker) with mild cheese sauce	½ cup	17.0
Mashed:		
(American Beauty)	½ cup	17.0
(Betty Crocker) *Buds*	½ cup	15.0
(French's) *Big Tate*	½ cup	16.0
(Pillsbury) *Hungry Jack,* flakes	½ cup	17.0
Scalloped:		
(Betty Crocker)	½ cup	19.0
(French's) *Big Tate*	½ cup	25.0
(Libby's) *Potato Classics*	¾ cup	24.0
Sour cream & chive (Betty Crocker)	½ cup	19.0
***POTATO PANCAKE MIX**		
(French's) *Big Tate*	3″ pancake	5.7
POTATO SALAD:		
Home recipe	½ cup	16.8
Canned (Nalley's):		
Regular	4-oz. serving	17.0
German style	4-oz. serving	18.2
POTATO STICK (Durkee) *O & C*	1½-oz. can	22.0
POTATO, STUFFED, BAKED, frozen (Green Giant) with chive topping	½ potato	27.0
POTATO TOPPERS (Libby's)	1 T.	4.0
POUND CAKE (See CAKE, Pound)		
PRESERVE OR JAM (Crosse & Blackwell)	1 T.	14.8
PRETZEL:		
(Bachman) regular or butter	1 oz.	21.0

Food and Description	Measure or Quantity	Carbohydrates (grams)
(Featherweight) unsalted	1 piece	1.3
(Nabisco) *Mister Salty*, Dutch	1 piece	11.0
(Rokeach) *Baldies*	1 oz.	20.0
PRODUCT 19, cereal (Kellogg's)	¾ cup	24.0
PRUNE:		
Canned:		
(Del Monte):		
Moist-Pak	2 oz.	33.4
Stewed, solids & liq.	4 oz.	31.2
(Featherweight) stewed, water pack	½ cup	35.0
(Sunsweet) stewed	½ cup	32.0
Dried:		
(Del Monte):		
Breakfast or medium	2 oz.	35.3
Jumbo	2 oz.	36.9
(Sunsweet) pitted	2 oz.	36.0
PRUNE JUICE:		
(Del Monte)	6 fl. oz.	33.0
(Mott's)	6 fl. oz.	34.0
(Sunsweet) regular or with pulp	6 fl. oz.	33.0
PRUNE NECTAR, canned (Mott's)	6 fl. oz.	25.0
PRUNE WHIP, home recipe	½ cup	49.8
PUDDING OR PIE FILLING:		
Canned, regular pack:		
Banana:		
(Del Monte) *Pudding Cup*	5-oz. container	30.1
(Hunt's) *Snack Pack*	5-oz. container	24.0
Butterscotch:		
(Del Monte) *Pudding Cup*	5-oz. container	30.8
(Hunt's) *Snack Pack*	5-oz. container	27.0
Chocolate:		
(Del Monte) *Pudding Cup*	5-oz. container	32.9
(Hunt's) *Snack Pack*	5-oz. container	28.0
Rice:		
(Comstock)	½ of 7½-oz. can	23.0
(Hunt's) *Snack Pack*	5-oz. container	27.0
(Menner's)	½ of 7½-oz. can	23.0
Tapioca:		
(Del Monte) *Pudding Cup*	5-oz. container	30.1
(Hunt's) *Snack Pack*	5-oz. container	23.0
Vanilla (Del Monte)	5-oz. container	32.1
Canned, dietetic pack (Sego) all flavors	4-oz. serving	39.0
Chilled, *Swiss Miss:*		
Butterscotch or Chocolate malt	4-oz. container	22.0

Food and Description	Measure or Quantity	Carbohydrates (grams)
Chocolate or vanilla	4-oz. container	25.0
Tapioca	4-oz. container	23.0
Frozen (Rich's):		
Banana	3-oz. container	19.3
Butterscotch	4½-oz. container	27.4
Chocolate	4½-oz. container	27.1
Vanilla	4½-oz. container	27.5
Mix, sweetened, regular & instant:		
Banana:		
*(Jello-O) cream:		
Regular	½-cup	26.7
Instant	½ cup	30.0
*(Royal):		
Regular	½ cup	27.0
Instant	½ cup	29.0
*Butter Pecan (Jell-O) instant	½ cup	29.1
Butterscotch:		
*(Jell-O) regular or instant	½ cup	30.0
*(My-T-Fine) regular	½ cup	28.0
*(Royal) instant	½ cup	29.0
Chocolate:		
*(Jell-O) regular	½ cup	28.8
*(My-T-Fine) regular	½ cup	27.0
*(Royal) instant	½ cup	35.0
Coconut:		
*(Jell-O) cream, regular	½ cup	24.4
*(Royal) instant	½ cup	30.0
Custard *(Royal) regular	½ cup	22.0
*Flan (Royal) regular	½ cup	22.0
Lemon:		
*(Jell-O) instant	½ cup	31.1
*(My-T-Fine) regular	½ cup	30.0
*(Royal) instant	½ cup	29.0
*Lime (Royal) Key Lime, regular	½ cup	30.0
*Pineapple (Jell-O) cream, regular	½ cup	30.4
Pistachio *(Royal) nut, instant	½ cup	30.0
*Raspberry (Salada) Danish Dessert	½ cup	32.0
*Rice, Jell-O Americana	½ cup	29.9
Tapioca:		
*Jell-O Americana, chocolate or vanilla	½ cup	27.8
*(My-T-Fine) vanilla	½ cup	28.0
*(Royal) vanilla	½ cup	27.0

Food and Description	Measure or Quantity	Carbohydrates (grams)
Vanilla:		
*(Jell-O) regular	½ cup	26.5
*(Jell-O) French, regular & instant	½ cup	30.0
*(My-T-Fine) regular	½ cup	28.0
*(Royal) instant	½ cup	29.0
*Mix, dietetic:		
Butterscotch:		
(D-Zerta)	½ cup	12.3
(Featherweight) artificially sweetened)	½ cup	9.0
Chocolate:		
(D-Zerta)	½ cup	11.5
(Estee)	½ cup	11.0
(Featherweight) artificially sweetened	½ cup	9.0
Lemon:		
(Dia-Mel)	½ cup	8.2
(Estee)	½ cup	26.6
Vanilla:		
(D-Zerta)	½ cup	12.7
(Estee)	½ cup	9.1
(Featherweight) artificially sweetened	½ cup	9.0
PUFFED RICE:		
(Malt-O-Meal)	1 cup	12.0
(Quaker)	1 cup	12.7
PUFFED WHEAT:		
(Malt-O-Meal)	1 cup	11.0
(Quaker)	1 cup	10.8
PUMPKIN, canned (Libby's)	½ cup	20.0
PUMPKIN SEED, in hull	1 oz.	3.2

Q

QUAIL, raw, meat & skin	4 oz.	0.
QUIK (Nestlé) chocolate or strawberry	1 tsp.	10.0
QUISP, cereal	1⅙ cups	23.1

R

RADISH	2 small radishes	3.5
RAISIN, dried:		
(Del Monte) golden	3 oz.	67.8
(Sun-Maid)	3 oz.	69.0
RAISINS, RICE & RYE, cereal		
(Kellogg's)	¾ cup	31.0
RALSTON, cereal	¼ cup	20.0
RASPBERRY:		
Fresh:		
Black, trimmed	½ cup	10.5
Red, trimmed	½ cup	9.8
Frozen (Birds Eye) quick thaw	5-oz. serving	37.0
RASPBERRY PRESERVE OR JAM:		
Sweetened (Smucker's)	1 T.	13.5
Dietetic (S&W) *Nutradiet*, red	1 T.	3.0
RASPBERRY SPREAD, low sugar		
(Smucker's)	1 T.	6.0
RAVIOLI:		
Canned, regular pack:		
(Franco-American):		
Beef, *RavioliOs*	7½-oz. serving	36.0
Cheese, in tomato sauce,		
RavioliOs	7½-oz. can	39.0
(Nalley's) beef	8-oz. serving	34.1
Canned, dietetic (Featherweight)		
beef, low sodium	8-oz. can	35.0
RELISH:		
Hamburger (Nalley's)	1 T.	4.1
Hot dog (Nalley's)	1 T.	4.8
Sweet (Smucker's)	1 T.	3.3
RENNET MIX (Junket):		
*Powder, any flavor, made with		
skim or whole milk	½ cup	16.0
Tablet	1 tablet	0.
RHINE WINE:		
(Great Western)	3 fl. oz.	2.9
(Inglenook) Navalle	3 fl. oz.	4.3
(Taylor)	3 fl. oz.	3.0
RHUBARB, cooked, sweetened	½ cup	43.2

Food and Description	*Measure or Quantity*	*Carbohydrates (grams)*
RICE:		
*Brown (Uncle Ben's) parboiled, with added butter	⅔ cup	26.4
*White:		
(Minute Rice) instant, no added butter	⅔ cup	27.4
(Uncle Ben's) parboiled	⅔ cup	23.3
(Success) long grain	½ cooking bag	23.0
*White & wild (Carolina)	½ cup	20.0
RICE, FRIED (See also RICE MIX):		
*Canned (La Choy)	½ oz. 11-oz. can	39.7
Frozen:		
(Birds Eye)	3.7 oz.	23.3
(La Choy) & pork	6-oz. serving	38.8
(Chun King)	5 oz.	24.0
***RICE, FRIED, SEASONING MIX** (Durkee)	1 cup	46.5
RICE KRINKLES, cereal (Post)	⅞ cup	25.9
RICE KRISPIES, cereal (Kellogg's)	1 cup	25.0
RICE MIX:		
Beef:		
*(Carolina) *Bake-It-Easy*	¼ of pkg.	23.0
(Minute-Rice)	½ cup	25.1
Rice-A-Roni	⅙ of 8-oz. pkg.	26.0
Chicken:		
*(Carolina) *Bake-It-Easy*	¼ of pkg.	23.0
Rice-A-Roni	⅕ of 8-oz. pkg.	33.2
*Fried (Minute Rice)	½ cup	25.2
*Long grain & wild (Uncle Ben's) with added butter	½ cup	20.6
*Oriental (Carolina) *Bake-It-Easy*	½ of pkg.	23.0
Spanish:		
*(Carolina) *Bake-It-Easy*	¼ of pkg.	23.0
*(Minute Rice)	½ cup	25.6
Rice-A-Roni	⅙ of 7½-oz. pkg.	25.9
RICE, SPANISH:		
Canned, regular pack:		
(Comstock)	½ of 7½-oz. can	27.0
(Libby's)	7½-oz. serving	27.5
Canned, dietetic (Featherweight)	7½ oz.	30.0
Frozen (Birds Eye)	3.7 oz.	26.1
RICE & VEGETABLES, frozen:		
(Birds Eye):		
French style	3.7 oz.	25.0
Peas & Mushroom	2⅓ oz.	23.1

Food and Description	Measure or Quantity	Carbohydrates (grams)
(Green Giant) *Rice Originals:*		
& broccoli in cheese sauce	½ cup	19.0
Festive	½ cup	24.0
Medley	½ cup	20.0
Verdi	½ cup	24.0
RICE WINE:		
Chinese, 20.7% alcohol	1 fl. oz.	1.1
Japanese, 10.6% alcohol	1 fl. oz.	13.1
RIESLING WINE, Grey (Inglenook)	3 fl. oz.	.7
ROCK & RYE (Mr. Boston)	1 fl. oz.	7.2
ROE, baked or broiled, cod & shad	4 oz.	2.2
ROLL OR BUN:		
Commercial type, non-frozen:		
Biscuit (Wonder)	1¼-oz. piece	17.0
Brown & serve (Wonder) *Gem Style*	1-oz. piece	13.1
Club (Pepperidge Farm)	1⅓-oz. piece	20.0
Crescent (Pepperidge Farm) butter	1-oz. piece	14.0
Croissant (Pepperidge Farm):		
Butter	2-oz. piece	19.0
Chocolate	2.4-oz. piece	25.0
Walnut	2-oz. piece	21.0
Dinner:		
Home Pride	1-oz. piece	14.2
(Pepperidge Farm)	1-oz. piece	10.0
(Wonder)	1¼-oz.	17.0
Finger, (Pepperidge Farm) sesame or poppy	.6-oz. piece	9.0
Frankfurter:		
(Pepperidge Farm)	1¾-oz. piece	18.0
(Wonder)	2-oz. piece	28.4
French:		
(Arnold) *Francisco*, Sourdough	1.1-oz. piece	16.0
(Pepperidge Farm):		
Small	1⅓-oz. piece	20.0
Large	3-oz. piece	44.0
Golden Twist (Pepperidge Farm)	1-oz. piece	20.0
Hamburger:		
(Arnold)	1.4-oz. piece	21.0
(Pepperidge Farm)	1½-oz. piece	23.0
Roman Meal	1.8-oz. piece	36.1
Hoggie (Wonder)	6-oz. piece	81.8
Honey (Hostess) glazed	3¾-oz. piece	52.2
Kaiser (Wonder)	6-oz. piece	81.8
Parkerhouse (Pepperidge Farm)	.6-oz. piece	9.0

Food and Description	Measure or Quantity	Carbohydrates (grams)
Party (Pepperidge Farm)	.4-oz. piece	22.0
Sandwich (Arnold) soft	1.3-oz. piece	18.0
Soft (Pepperidge Farm)	1¼-oz. piece	18.0
Frozen:		
Apple crunch (Sara Lee)	1-oz. piece	13.5
Caramel pecan (Sara Lee)	1.3-oz. piece	17.4
Cinnamon (Sara Lee)	.9-oz. piece	13.9
Croissant (Sara Lee)	.9-oz. piece	11.2
Crumb (Sara Lee):		
Blueberry	1¾-oz. piece	26.8
French	1¾-oz. piece	28.9
Danish (Sara Lee):		
Apple	1.3-oz. piece	17.4
Apple Country	1.8-oz. piece	22.9
Cheese	1.3-oz. piece	13.9
Cheese Country	1½-oz.	
Cherry	1.3-oz. piece	16.4
Cinnamon Raisin	1.3-oz. piece	17.3
Pecan	1.3-oz. piece	18.3
Honey:		
(Morton):		
Regular	2½-oz. piece	30.7
Mini	1.3-oz. piece	17.7
(Sara Lee)	1-oz. piece	15.2
ROLL OR BUN DOUGH:		
*Frozen (Rich's):		
Cinnamon	2¼-oz. roll	32.8
Frankfurter	1 roll	24.9
Hamburger, regular	1 roll	25.0
Onion, regular	1 roll	29.1
Parkerhouse	1 roll	13.4
Refrigerated (Pillsbury):		
Cinnamon with icing, *Ballard*	1 piece	17.0
Cinnamon raisin, danish	1 piece	20.0
Crescent	1 piece	24.0
White, Bakery Style	1 piece	18.0
*ROLL MIX, HOT (Pillsbury)	1 piece	17.0
ROMAN MEAL CEREAL	⅓ cup	20.0
ROSEMARY LEAVES (French's)	1 tsp.	.8
ROSE WINE:		
(Great Western)	3 fl. oz.	2.4
(Inglenook) Gamay or Vintage	3 fl. oz.	.5
(Paul Masson):		
Regular, 11.8% alcohol	3 fl. oz.	4.2

Food and Description	Measure or Quantity	Carbohydrates (grams)
Light, 7.1% alcohol	3 fl. oz.	3.2
RUTABAGA:		
Canned (Sunshine) solids & liq.	½ cup	6.9
Frozen (Southland)	4 oz.	13.0

S

Food and Description	Measure or Quantity	Carbohydrates (grams)
SAFFLOWER SEED in hull	¼ lb.	7.2
SAGE (French's)	1 tsp.	.6
SAKE WINE	1 fl. oz.	1.4
SALAD CRUNCHIES (Libby's)	1 T.	4.0
SALAD DRESSING:		
Regular:		
Bacon (Seven Seas) creamy	1 T.	1.0
Bleu or blue cheese:		
(Bernstein) Danish	1 T.	.6
(Wish-Bone) chunky	1 T.	1.0
Caesar (Wish-Bone)	1 T.	1.0
Capri (Seven Seas)	1 T.	3.0
Cucumber (Wish-Bone)	1 T.	2.0
French:		
(Bernstein's) creamy	1 T.	2.1
(Pfeiffer)	1 T.	3.5
(Seven Seas) creamy	1 T.	2.0
(Wish-Bone) deluxe or Sweet 'n Spicy	1 T.	3.0
Garlic (Wish-Bone) creamy	1 T.	2.0
Green Goddess:		
(Seven Seas)	1 T.	0.
(Wish-Bone)	1 T.	1.0
Italian:		
(Bernstein's)	1 T.	.8
(Seven Seas)	1 T.	1.0
(Wish-Bone) regular or robusto	1 T.	1.0
Louis Dressing (Nalley's)	1 T.	1.8
Onion 'N Chive (Seven Seas) creamy	1 T.	1.0
Red wine vinegar & oil (Seven Seas)	1 T.	1.0
Roquefort:		
(Bernstein's)	1 T.	.8
(Marie's)	1 T.	1.1
Russian:		
(Pfeiffer)	1 T.	4.0

Food and Description	Measure or Quantity	Carbohydrates (grams)
(Seven Seas) creamy	1 T.	1.0
(Wish-Bone)	1 T.	7.0
Spin Blend (Hellmann's)	1 T.	2.6
Thousand Island:		
(Pfeiffer)	1 T.	4.0
(Wish-Bone)	1 T.	3.0
Vinaigrette (Bernstein's) French	1 T.	.2
Dietetic:		
Bleu or blue cheese:		
(Featherweight) imitation	1 T.	1.0
(Tillie Lewis) *Tasti-Diet*	1 T.	<1.0
(Wish-Bone) chunky	1 T.	3.0
Caesar:		
(Estee) garlic	1 T.	1.0
(Featherweight) creamy	1 T.	2.0
(Pfeiffer)	1 T.	
Cucumber (Featherweight) creamy	1 T.	0.
Cucumber & onion (Featherweight) creamy	1 T.	1.0
French:		
(Featherweight)	1 T.	0.
(Tillie Lewis) *Tasti-Diet*	1 T.	<1.0
(Walden Farms) chunky	1 T.	3.0
(Wish-Bone)	1 T.	4.0
Herb & Spice (Featherweight)	1 T.	1.0
Italian:		
(Estee) spicy	1 T.	1.0
(Featherweight)	1 T.	1.0
(Tillie Lewis) *Tasti-Diet*	1 T.	0.
(Weight Watchers)	1 T.	2.0
(Wish-Bone)	1 T.	3.0
Onion n'Chive (Wish-Bone)	1 T.	1.0
Red wine/vinegar (Featherweight)	1 T.	1.0
Russian:		
(Featherweight) creamy	1 T.	1.0
(Tillie Lewis) *Tasti-Diet*	1 T.	<1.0
(Weight Watchers)	1 T.	2.0
(Wish-Bone)	1 T.	5.0
Thousand Island:		
(Pfeiffer)	1 T.	2.8
(Walden Farms)	1 T.	3.0
(Weight Watchers)	1 T.	2.0
(Wish-Bone)	1 T.	3.0
2-Calorie Low Sodium		
(Featherweight)	1 T.	0.

Food and Description	Measure or Quantity	Carbohydrates (grams)
Whipped (Tillie Lewis) *Tasti-Diet*	1 T.	1.0
SALAD DRESSING MIX:		
*Regular (Good Seasons):		
Bleu or blue cheese	1 T.	.3
Buttermilk Farm Style	1 T.	1.3
Farm Style	1 T.	.6
French:		
Regular	1 T.	2.9
Old fashioned	1 T.	.5
Garlic, regular or cheese	1 T.	.5
Italian, regular or zesty	1 T.	.7
Onion	1 T.	.6
Dietetic:		
*Blue cheese (Weight Watchers)	1 T.	1.0
*French (Weight Watchers)	1 T.	1.0
Italian:		
*(Good Seasons)	1 T.	1.8
*(Weight Watchers):		
Regular	1 T.	0.
Creamy	1 T.	1.0
*Russian (Weight Watchers)	1 T.	1.0
*Thousand Island (Weight Watchers)	1 T.	1.0
SALAMI:		
(Hormel):		
Cotto	1-oz. slice	0.
Genoa, sliced	1-oz. slice	.6
(Oscar Mayer):		
For beer	.8-oz. slice	.4
For beer, beef	.8-oz. slice	.2
Cotto	.8-oz. slice	.4
Hard	.3-oz. slice	.2
(Swift) Genoa	1-oz. serving	.3
(Vienna) beef	1-oz. serving	.8
SALISBURY STEAK:		
Canned (Morton House)	6½-oz. serving	7.0
Frozen:		
(Banquet):		
Buffet Supper	2-lb. pkg.	48.2
Man Pleaser	19-oz. dinner	71.7
(Green Giant) with gravy	7-oz. serving	13.9
(Stouffer's) with onion gravy	12 oz.	40.0
(Swanson):		
Regular, with gravy	10-oz. entree	14.0
Hungry Man	17-oz. dinner	63.0
3-course	16-oz. dinner	50.0

Food and Description	Measure or Quantity	Carbohydrates (grams)
TV Brand	11½-oz. dinner	43.0
SALMON	any quantity	0.
SALMON, SMOKED (Vita):		
Lox, drained	4-oz. jar	.2
Nova, drained	4-oz. can	1.0
SALT:		
Table (Morton) regular or Lite	1 tsp.	0.
Substitute:		
(Adolph's):		
Plain	1 tsp.	Tr.
Seasoned	1 tsp.	1.1
(Morton) plain	1 tsp.	Tr.
SANDWICH SPREAD:		
(Hellmann's)	1 T.	2.2
(Oscar Mayer)	1-oz. serving	3.2
SANGRIA (Taylor)	3 fl. oz.	10.8
SARDINE, canned:		
Atlantic (Del Monte) with tomato sauce	7½-oz. can	3.8
Imported (Underwood) in mustard or tomato sauce	3¾-oz. can	<1.0
Norwegian, *King Oscar Brand:*		
In mustard or tomato sauce	3¾-oz. can	2.0
In oil, drained	3-oz. can	1.0
SAUCE:		
Regular pack:		
A-1	1 T.	3.1
Barbecue:		
Chris & Pitt's	1 T.	4.0
(French's) regular or smoky	1 T.	5.0
(Gold's)	1 T.	3.9
Open Pit (General Foods) hickory smoke	1 T.	5.5
Chili (See CHILI SAUCE)		
Cocktail:		
(Gold's)	1 T.	7.5
(Nalley's)	1-oz. serving	14.2
Escoffier Sauce Diable	1 T.	4.3
Escoffier Sauce Robert	1 T.	5.1
Famous Sauce	1 T.	2.2
Hot, *Frank's*	1 tsp.	0.
Italian:		
(Contadina)	4 fl. oz.	10.5
(Ragu) red cooking	3½-oz. serving	6.0
Salsa Mexicana (Contadina)	4 fl. oz.	6.8
Salsa Picante (Del Monte)	¼ cup	3.0

112

Food and Description	Measure or Quantity	Carbohydrates (grams)
Salsa Roja (Del Monte)	¼ cup	4.0
Seafood cocktail (Del Monte)	1 T.	4.9
Soy:		
(Gold's)	1 T.	1.0
(Kikkoman)	1 T.	.9
(La Choy)	1 T.	.9
Spare rib (Gold's)	1 T.	11.7
Steak (Dawn Fresh) with mushrooms	1-oz. serving	1.7
Steak Supreme	1 T.	5.1
Sweet & sour:		
(Contadina)	1 oz.	7.6
(La Choy)	1 oz.	12.6
Taco:		
(Del Monte) hot or mild	¼ cup	4.0
Old El Paso	1-oz. serving	2.3
(Ortega)	1 T.	5.1
Tartar:		
(Hellmann's)	1 T.	.2
(Nalley's)	1 T.	.3
Teriyaki (Kikkoman)	1 T.	3.1
V-8	1 oz. serving	6.0
White, medium	¼ cup	5.6
Worcestershire:		
(French's) regular or smoky	1 T.	2.0
(Gold's)	1 T.	3.3
SAUCE MIX:		
Regular:		
A la King (Durkee)	1-oz. pkg.	14.0
*Cheese:		
(Durkee)	½ cup	9.5
(French's)	½ cup	14.0
Hollandaise:		
(Durkee)	1-oz. pkg.	11.0
*(French's)	1 T.	.7
Sour cream:		
*(Durkee)	⅔ cup	15.0
*(French's)	2½ T.	5.0
*Sweet & sour (Durkee)	1 cup	45.0
*Teriyaki (French's)	1 T.	3.5
*White (Durkee)	1 cup	41.0
*Dietetic (Weight Watchers) lemon butter	1 T.	1.0
SAUERKRAUT:		
(Claussen) drained	½ cup	2.8
(Del Monte) solids & liq.	1 cup	10.6
(Silver Floss) solids & liq.	½ cup	5.0

113

Food and Description	Measure or Quantity	Carbohydrates (grams)
SAUSAGE:		
Brown 'n Serve (Swift) original	.8-oz. link	.5
Italian style (Best's Kosher; Oscherwitz)	3-oz. link	.7
Polish-style:		
(Best's Kosher; Oscherwitz)	3-oz. link	1.8
(Vienna) beef	3-oz. link	1.3
Pork:		
*(Hormel) *Little Sizzlers*	1 link	<1.0
(Jimmy Dean)	2-oz. serving	Tr.
*(Oscar Mayer) *Little Friers*	.6-oz. link	.2
Smoked:		
(Eckrich) beef, *Smok-Y-Links*	.8-oz. link	1.0
(Hormel) pork	3-oz. serving	.7
(Oscar Mayer) beef	1½-oz. link	.9
(Vienna)	2½-oz. serving	.9
*Turkey (Louis Rich) links or tube	1-oz. serving	<1.0
SAUSAGE SANDWICH, frozen (Stouffer's)	8¼ oz.	40.0
SAUTERNE:		
(Great Western)	3 fl. oz.	4.5
(Taylor)	3 fl. oz.	4.8
SCALLOP:		
Frozen (Mrs. Paul's):		
Breaded & fried	3½-oz. serving	24.1
With butter & cheese	7-oz. pkg.	11.2
SCHAV SOUP (Gold's)	8-oz. serving	2.1
SCHNAPPS, APPLE (Mr. Boston)	1 fl. oz.	8.0
SCHNAPPS, PEPPERMINT (Mr. Boston)	1 fl. oz.	8.0
SCREWDRIVER COCKTAIL:		
Canned (Mr. Boston) 12½% alcohol	3 fl. oz.	12.0
Mix, dry (Bar-Tender's)	1 serving	17.4
SEAFOOD PLATTER, frozen (Mrs. Paul's) breaded, fried	4½-oz. serving	28.5
SEGO DIET FOOD, canned:		
Milk chocolate, very chocolate, very chocolate coconut	10 fl. oz.	39.0
Very butterscotch, very cherry vanilla or very vanilla	10 fl. oz.	34.0
Canned, any flavor	10-fl.-oz. can	
SELTZER (Canada Dry)	any quantity	0.
SERUTAN:		
Toasted granules	1 tsp.	1.3
Fruit-flavored powder	1 tsp.	1.5

114

Food and Description	Measure or Quantity	Carbohydrates (grams)
SESAME SEEDS (French's)	1 tsp.	.9
SHAD, CREOLE	4-oz. serving	1.8
SHAKE 'N BAKE:		
Chicken, original	1 pkg.	41.6
Crispy country mild	1 pkg.	40.4
Fish	2-oz. pkg.	17.0
Italian	1 pkg.	41.2
Pork:		
Original	1 pkg.	48.1
Barbecue	1 pkg.	59.2
SHERBERT:		
(Baskin-Robbins):		
Daiquiri Ice	1 scoop	20.9
Orange	1 scoop	20.9
(Meadow Gold) orange	¼ pint	26.0
SHERRY:		
Cocktail (Gold Seal)	3 fl. oz.	1.6
Cream:		
(Great Western) Solera	3 fl. oz.	12.2
(Taylor)	3 fl. oz.	13.2
Dry:		
(Italian Swiss Colony) *Gold Medal*	3 fl. oz.	1.7
(Williams & Humbert)	3 fl. oz.	4.5
Dry Sack (Williams & Humbert)	3 fl. oz.	4.5
SHREDDED WHEAT:		
(Nabisco):		
Regular size	¾-oz. biscuit	19.0
Spoon Size	⅔ cup	23.0
(Quaker)	1 biscuit	11.0
SHRIMP:		
Raw, meat only	4 oz.	1.7
Canned:		
(Bumble Bee) solids & liq.	4½-oz. can	.9
(Icy Point) cocktail	4½-oz. can	.8
Frozen (Mrs. Paul's) fried	3-oz. serving	16.8
SHRIMP DINNER, frozen (Van de Kamp's)	10-oz. dinner	40.0
SHRIMP PUFF (Durkee)	1 piece	3.0
SLENDER (Carnation):		
Bar:		
Chocolate, chocolate chip	1 bar	13.0
All other flavors	1 bar	12.5
Dry	1 packet	21.0
Liquid	10-fl.-oz. can	34.0
SLOPPY HOT DOG SEASONING MIX (French's)	1½-oz. pkg.	28.0

Food and Description	Measure or Quantity	Carbohydrates (grams)
SLOPPY JOE:		
Canned:		
(Hormel) *Short Orders*	7½-oz. can	15.0
(Libby's):		
Beef	⅓ cup	7.0
Pork	⅓ cup	6.0
(Morton House) beef	5-oz. serving	19.0
Frozen (Banquet) *Cookin' Bag*	5-oz. bag	11.2
SLOPPY JOE SEASONING MIX:		
*(Durkee):		
Regular flavor	1¼ cups	30.0
Pizza flavor	1¼ cups	26.0
(French's)	1½-oz. pkg.	32.0
SNACK BAR (Pepperidge Farm):		
Apple nut	1.7-oz. piece	33.0
Apricot-raspberry or blueberry	1.7-oz. piece	36.0
Brownie nut or date nut	1½-oz. piece	30.0
Chocolate chip or coconut		
macaroon	1½-oz. piece	28.0
Raisin spice	1½-oz. piece	31.0
SNO BALL (Hostess)	1 cake	27.3
SOAVE WINE (Antinori)	3 fl. oz.	6.3
SOFT DRINK:		
Sweetened:		
Birch beer (Canada Dry)	6 fl. oz.	21.0
Bitter lemon:		
(Canada Dry)	6 fl. oz.	19.5
(Schweppes)	6 fl. oz.	20.8
Bubble Up	6 fl. oz.	18.4
Cactus Cooler (Canada Dry)	6 fl. oz.	21.8
Cherry:		
(Canada Dry) wild	6 fl. oz.	24.0
(Shasta) black	6 fl. oz.	21.5
Chocolate (Yoo-Hoo)	6 fl. oz.	24.1
Club (any brand)	6 fl. oz.	0.
Cola:		
Coca-Cola:		
Regular	6 fl. oz.	19.0
Caffeine-free	6 fl. oz.	20.0
Jamaica (Canada Dry)	6 fl. oz.	20.2
Pepsi-Cola, regular or *Pepsi Free*	6 fl. oz.	19.8
(Royal Crown)	6 fl. oz.	19.4
(Shasta)	6 fl. oz.	19.5
Collins mix (Canada Dry)	6 fl. oz.	15.0

Food and Description	Measure or Quantity	Carbohydrates (grams)
Cream:		
(Canada Dry) vanilla	6 fl. oz.	24.0
(Schweppes) red	6 fl. oz.	21.3
(Shasta)	6 fl. oz.	20.5
Dr. Pepper	6 fl. oz.	19.4
Fruit Punch:		
(Nehi)	6 fl. oz.	22.8
(Shasta)	6 fl. oz.	23.0
Ginger ale:		
(Canada Dry) regular	6 fl. oz.	15.8
(Fanta)	6 fl. oz.	16.0
(Schweppes)	6 fl. oz.	16.3
Ginger beer (Schweppes)	6 fl. oz.	16.8
Grape:		
(Canada Dry) concord	6 fl. oz.	24.0
(Hi-C)	6 fl. oz.	20.0
(Nehi)	6 fl. oz.	21.8
(Schweppes)	6 fl. oz.	23.8
(Welch's) sparkling	6 fl. oz.	23.0
Half & half (Canada Dry)	6 fl. oz.	19.5
Hi-Spot (Canada Dry)	6 fl. oz.	18.7
Island Lime (Canada Dry)	6 fl. oz.	24.8
Lemon-lime (Shasta)	6 fl. oz.	19.0
Mello Yello	6 fl. oz.	22.0
Mountain Dew	6 fl. oz.	22.2
Mr. PiBB	6 fl. oz.	19.0
Orange:		
(Canada Dry) *Sunripe*	6 fl. oz.	24.7
(Fanta)	6 fl. oz.	23.0
(Shasta)	6 fl. oz.	23.5
(Sunkist)	6 fl. oz.	7.6
(Welch's)	6 fl. oz.	23.5
Peach (Nehi)	6 fl. oz.	23.0
Pineapple (Canada Dry)	6 fl. oz.	19.5
Quinine or Tonic Water:		
(Canada Dry)	6 fl. oz.	16.5
(Schweppes)	6 fl. oz.	16.5
(Shasta)	6 fl. oz.	16.0
Rondo (Schweppes)	6 fl. oz.	19.5
Root Beer:		
Barrelhead (Canada Dry)	6 fl. oz.	19.5
(Dad's)	6 fl. oz.	20.7
(Nehi)	6 fl. oz.	21.8
On Tap	6 fl. oz.	20.4
Rooti (Canada Dry)	6 fl. oz.	19.5
(Shasta) draft	6 fl. oz.	20.5

Food and Description	Measure or Quantity	Carbohydrates (grams)
Seven-Up	6 fl. oz.	18.1
Sprite	6 fl. oz.	18.0
Strawberry:		
(Canada Dry) California	6 fl. oz.	22.5
(Shasta)	6 fl. oz.	19.5
(Welch's)	6 fl. oz.	23.5
Tahitian Treat (Canada Dry)	6 fl. oz.	24.0
Teem	6 fl. oz.	18.6
Upper 10 (Royal Crown)	6 fl. oz.	19.0
Vanilla:		
Whiskey sour (Canada Dry)	6 fl. oz.	16.5
Wink (Canada Dry)	6 fl. oz.	22.5
Dietetic or low calorie:		
Bubble Up	6 fl. oz.	.2
Cherry:		
(No-Cal) black	6 fl. oz.	Tr.
(Shasta) black	6 fl. oz.	Tr.
Chocolate (No-Cal)	6 fl. oz.	Tr.
Coffee (No-Cal)	6 fl. oz.	Tr.
Cola:		
(Canada Dry)	6 fl. oz.	0.
Coca-Cola, regular or caffeine free	6 fl. oz.	.1
Diet-Rite	6 fl. oz.	Tr.
(No-Cal)	6 fl. oz.	0.
Pepsi, diet, Free or light	6 fl. oz.	Tr.
(Shasta) regular or cherry	6 fl. oz.	Tr.
Cream:		
(No-Cal)	6 fl. oz.	0.
(Shasta)	6 fl. oz.	Tr.
Dr. Pepper	6 fl. oz.	.4
Fresca	6 fl. oz.	Tr.
Ginger Ale:		
(Canada Dry)	6 fl. oz.	Tr.
(No-Cal)	6 fl. oz.	Tr.
(Shasta)	6 fl. oz.	Tr.
Grape (Shasta)	6 fl. oz.	Tr.
Grapefruit (Shasta)	6 fl. oz.	.2
Mr. PiBB	6 fl. oz.	.2
Orange:		
(No-Cal)	6 fl. oz.	Tr.
(Shasta)	6 fl. oz.	Tr.
Tab	6 fl. oz.	Tr.
Quinine or Tonic (No-Cal)	6 fl. oz.	Tr.
RC 100 (Royal Crown)	6 fl. oz.	Tr.

Food and Description	Measure or Quantity	Carbohydrates (grams)
Root Beer:		
Barrelhead (Canada Dry)	6 fl. oz.	Tr.
(Dad's)	6 fl. oz.	.2
(No-Cal)	6 fl. oz.	0.
(Ramblin')	6 fl. oz.	.2
(Shasta) draft	6 fl. oz.	Tr.
Seven-Up	6 fl. oz.	Tr.
Sprite	6 fl. oz.	Tr.
Strawberry (Shasta)	6 fl. oz.	Tr.
Tab	6 fl. oz.	.2
SOLE, frozen:		
(Mrs. Paul's) fillets, with lemon butter	4½-oz. serving	9.7
(Van de Kamp's) batter dipped, french fried	1 piece	12.0
(Weight Watchers) in lemon sauce	9¼-oz. meal	17.0
SOUP:		
Canned, regular pack:		
*Asparagus (Campbell) condensed, cream of	8 oz.	11.0
Bean:		
(Campbell):		
Chunky, with ham, old fashioned	11-oz. can	37.0
*Condensed, with bacon	8 oz.	21.0
*Semi-condensed, *Soup For One,* with ham	11 oz.	31.0
(Grandma Brown's)	8 oz.	29.1
Bean, black:		
*(Campbell) condensed	8 oz.	17.0
(Crosse & Blackwell)	6½ oz.	18.0
Beef:		
(Campbell):		
Chunky:		
Regular	10 ¾-oz. can	23.0
With noodles	10 ¾-oz. can	28.0
*Condensed:		
Regular	8 oz.	10.0
Broth:		
Plain	8 oz.	1.0
& barley	8 oz.	10.0
& noodles	8 oz.	9.0
Consomme	8 oz.	2.0
Mushroom	8 oz.	6.0
Noodle	8 oz.	7.0
Teriyaki	8 oz.	9.0

Food and Description	Measure or Quantity	Carbohydrates (grams)
(College Inn) broth	1 cup	1.0
(Swanson)	7½-oz. can	1.0
Celery:		
*(Campbell) condensed, cream of	8 oz.	8.0
*(Rokeach) condensed:		
Prepared with milk	10 oz.	19.0
Prepared with water	10 oz.	12.0
*Cheddar cheese (Campbell)	8 oz.	10.0
Chicken:		
(Campbell):		
Chunky:		
Regular	10 ¾-oz. can	20.0
Old fashioned	10 ¾-oz. can	21.0
& rice	19-oz. can	30.0
Vegetable	19-oz. can	38.0
*Condensed:		
Alphabet	8 oz.	10.0
Broth:		
Plain	8 oz.	3.0
& rice	8 oz.	8.0
Cream of	8 oz.	9.0
Gumbo	8 oz.	8.0
Mushroom, creamy	8 oz.	9.0
NoodleOs	8 oz.	9.0
Oriental	8 oz.	5.0
& rice	8 oz.	7.0
Vegetable	8 oz.	8.0
*Semi-condensed, *Soup For One:*		
& noodles, golden	11 oz.	14.0
Vegetable, full flavored	11 oz.	13.0
(College Inn) broth	1 cup	0.
(Swanson) broth	7¼-oz. can	3.0
Chili beef (Campbell):		
Chunky	11-oz. can	37.0
*Condensed	8 oz.	17.0
Chowder:		
Beef'n vegetable (Hormel)	7½-oz. can	15.0
Chicken'n corn (Hormel)	7½-oz. can	15.0
Clam:		
Manhattan style:		
(Campbell):		
Chunky	18-oz. can	44.0
*Condensed	8 oz.	11.0
(Crosse & Blackwell)	6½ oz.	9.0

Food and Description	Measure or Quantity	Carbohydrates (grams)
New England style:		
*(Campbell):		
Condensed:		
Made with milk	8 oz.	17.0
Made with water	8 oz.	11.0
Semi-condensed, *Soup for One:*		
Made with milk	11 oz.	23.0
Made with water	11 oz.	18.0
(Crosse & Blackwell)	6½-oz.	14.0
Ham'n potato (Hormel)	7½-oz. can	14.0
Consomme madrilene (Crosse & Blackwell)	6½ oz.	5.0
Crab (Crosse & Blackwell)	6½ oz.	8.0
Gazpacho:		
*(Campbell's) condensed	8 oz.	9.0
(Crosse & Blackwell)	6½ oz.	1.0
Ham'n butter bean (Campbell) *Chunky*	10 ¾-oz. can	33.0
Lentil (Crosse & Blackwell) with ham	6½ oz.	13.0
*Meatball alphabet (Campbell) condensed	8 oz.	12.0
Mexicali bean (Campbell) *Chunky*	19½-oz. can	70.0
Minestrone:		
(Campbell):		
Chunky	18-oz. can	42.0
*Condensed	8 oz.	11.0
(Crosse & Blackwell)	6½-oz.	18.0
Mushroom:		
*(Campbell):		
Condensed:		
Cream of	8 oz.	9.0
Golden	8 oz.	10.0
Semi-condensed, *Soup For One,* cream of, savory	11 oz.	15.0
(Crosse & Blackwell) cream of, bisque	6½ oz.	8.0
*(Rokeach) cream of:		
Prepared with milk	10 oz.	20.0
Prepared with water	10 oz.	13.0
*Mushroom barley (Campbell's)	8 oz.	12.0
*Noodle (Campbell):		
Curley noodle with chicken	8 oz.	9.0
& ground beef	8 oz.	10.0

Food and Description	Measure or Quantity	Carbohydrates (grams)
*Onion (Campbell):		
Regular	8 oz.	9.0
Cream of:		
Made with water	8 oz.	12.0
Made with water & milk	8 oz.	15.0
*Oyster stew (Campbell):		
Made with milk	8 oz.	10.0
Made with water	8 oz.	5.0
*Pea, green (Campbell)	8 oz.	25.0
Pea, split:		
(Campbell):		
Chunky, with ham	18-oz. can	58.0
*Condensed, with ham &		
bacon	8 oz.	24.0
(Grandma Brown's)	8 oz.	28.2
*Pepper pot (Campbell)	8 oz.	9.0
*Potato (Campbell) cream of:		
Made with water	8 oz.	11.0
Made with water & milk	8 oz.	14.0
*Scotch broth (Campbell)	8 oz.	9.0
Shrimp:		
*(Campbell) condensed, cream of:		
Made with milk	8 oz.	22.0
Made with water	8 oz.	8.0
(Crosse & Blackwell) cream of	6½ oz.	7.0
Sirloin burger (Campbell) Chunky	19-oz. can	40.0
Steak & potato (Campbell) Chunky	19-oz. can	42.0
Tomato:		
*(Campbell):		
Condensed:		
Regular:		
Made with milk	8 oz.	22.0
Made with water	8 oz.	17.0
Bisque	8 oz.	23.0
& rice, old fashioned	8 oz.	22.0
Semi-condensed, Soup For One, Royale	11 oz.	35.0
*(Rokeach):		
Made with milk	10 oz.	27.0
Made with water	10 oz.	20.0
Turkey (Campbell):		
Chunky	18 ¾-oz. can	36.0
*Condensed:		
Noodle	8 oz.	8.0
Vegetable	8 oz.	8.0

Food and Description	Measure or Quantity	Carbohydrates (grams)
Vegetable:		
(Campbell):		
Chunky:		
Regular	19-oz. can	42.0
Beef, old fashioned	19-oz. can	18.0
Mediterranean	19-oz. can	48.0
*Condensed:		
Regular	8 oz.	11.0
Beef	8 oz.	8.0
Vegetarian	8 oz.	12.0
*Semi-condensed, *Soup For One:*		
Barley, with beef	11 oz.	20.0
Old world	11 oz.	18.0
*(Rokeach) vegetarian	10 oz.	15.0
Vichyssoise (Crosse & Blackwell) cream of	6½ oz.	5.0
*Won ton (Campbell)	8 oz.	5.0
Canned, dietetic pack:		
Beef:		
(Campbell) & mushroom, low sodium	10 ¾-oz. can	23.0
(Dia-Mel) & noodle	8 oz.	5.0
Chicken:		
(Campbell) low sodium:		
Chunky	7½-oz. can	14.0
With noodles	10 ¾-oz. can	19.0
Vegetable	10 ¾-oz. can	21.0
*(Dia-Mel) broth	8 oz.	1.0
Corn (Campbell) low sodium	10 ¾-oz. can	31.0
Mushroom (Campbell) cream of, low sodium	7¼-oz. can	10.0
Pea, green (Campbell) low sodium	7½-oz. can	23.0
Pea, split (Campbell) low sodium	10 ¾-oz. can	35.0
Tomato (Campbell) low sodium:		
Regular	7¼-oz. can	24.0
With tomato pieces	10½-oz. can	32.0
Turkey (Campbell) & noodle, low sodium	7¼-oz. can	8.0
Vegetable (Campbell) low sodium:		
Regular	7¼-oz. can	15.0
Chunky	10 ¾-oz. can	22.0
Frozen:		
*Barley & mushroom (Mother's Own)	8 oz.	8.0

Food and Description	Measure or Quantity	Carbohydrates (grams)
Chowder, Clam, New England style (Stouffer's)	8 oz.	19.0
Pea, split:		
*(Mother's Own)	8 oz.	20.0
(Stouffer's)	8¼ oz.	27.0
Spinach (Stouffer's) cream of	8 oz.	17.0
*Vegetable (Mother's Own)	8 oz.	Tr.
*Won ton (La Choy)	1 cup	12.3
Mix, regular:		
Beef:		
*Carmel Kosher	6 fl. oz.	1.8
*(Lipton):		
Cup-A-Soup, regular and noodle	6 fl. oz.	8.0
Lots-A-Noodles	7 fl. oz.	21.0
*(Weight Watchers) broth	6 fl. oz.	1.0
*Chicken:		
Carmel Kosher	6 fl. oz.	1.8
(Lipton):		
Regular	8 fl. oz.	8.0
Cup-A-Broth	6 fl. oz.	4.0
Cup-A-Soup:		
Regular:		
Cream of	6 fl. oz.	9.0
& rice	6 fl. oz.	7.0
& vegetable	6 fl. oz.	7.0
Country style:		
Hearty	6 fl. oz.	11.0
Supreme	6 fl. oz.	11.0
Lots-A-Noodles	7 fl. oz.	23.0
Noodle Soup:		
With chicken broth	8 fl. oz.	8.0
With chicken meat	8 fl. oz.	1.0
Giggle Noodle	8 fl. oz.	12.0
Ripple Noodle	8 fl. oz.	12.0
*Mushroom:		
Carmel Kosher	6 fl. oz.	2.0
(Lipton):		
Regular:		
Beef	8 fl. oz.	7.0
Onion	8 fl. oz.	6.0
Cup-A-Soup, cream of	6 fl. oz.	10.0
*Onion:		
Carmel Kosher	6 fl. oz.	2.4

Food and Description	Measure or Quantity	Carbohydrates (grams)
(Lipton):		
Regular:		
Plain	8 fl. oz.	6.0
Beefy	8 fl. oz.	4.0
Cup-A-Soup	6 fl. oz.	5.0
*Oriental (Lipton) *Cup-A-Soup*,		
Lots-A-Noodles	7 fl. oz.	20.0
*Pea, green (Lipton) *Cup-A-Soup*	6 fl. oz.	16.0
*Pea, Virginia (Lipton)		
Cup-A-Soup, Country Style	6 fl. oz.	18.0
*Tomato (Lipton) *Cup-A-Soup*	6 fl. oz.	17.0
*Vegetable (Lipton):		
Regular:		
Beef	8 fl. oz.	7.0
Country	8 fl. oz.	14.0
Cup-A-Soup:		
Regular:		
Beef	6 fl. oz.	8.0
Spring	6 fl. oz.	7.0
Country Style, harvest	6 fl. oz.	20.0
Lots-A-Noodles, garden	7 fl. oz.	23.0
(Southland) frozen	⅕ of 16-oz. pkg.	12.0
SOUP GREENS (Durkee)	2½-oz. jar	43.0
SOUTHERN COMFORT:		
80 proof	1 fl. oz.	3.4
86 proof or 100 proof	1 fl. oz.	3.5
SOYBEAN CURD or TOFU	2¾" × 1½" × 1"cake	2.9
SPAGHETTI:		
Cooked:		
8-10 minutes, "al dente"	1 cup	43.9
14-20 minutes, tender	1 cup	32.2
Canned:		
(Franco-American):		
With little meatballs in tomato		
sauce	7⅜-oz. can	22.0
With meatballs in tomato		
sauce, *SpaghettiOs*	7⅜-oz. can	25.0
In meat sauce	7½-oz. can	26.0
With sliced franks in tomato		
sauce, *SpaghettiOs*	7⅜-oz. can	26.0
In tomato sauce with cheese	7⅜-oz. can	36.0
(Hormel) *Short Orders*, & meat-balls in tomato sauce	7½-oz. can	24.0
Dietetic (Featherweight) & meatballs	7½-oz. serving	28.0

Food and Description	Measure or Quantity	Carbohydrates (grams)
Frozen:		
(Banquet):		
Buffet Supper, & meatballs	2-lb-pkg.	129.1
Dinner, & meatballs	11½-oz. dinner	62.9
(Green Giant) & meatballs in tomato sauce	9-oz. entree	53.9
(Stouffer) & meat sauce	14-oz. pkg.	62.0
(Swanson) *TV Brand*	12½-oz. dinner	46.0
SPAGHETTI SAUCE:		
Canned, regular pack:		
Marinara:		
(Prince)	4-oz. serving	12.4
(Ragu)	5-oz. serving	15.0
Meat or meat flavored:		
(Prego)	4-oz. serving	22.0
(Prince)	½ cup	11.0
(Ragu)	5-oz. serving	14.0
Meatless or plain:		
(Hain)	4-oz. serving	14.2
(Prego)	4-oz. serving	22.0
(Prince)	½ cup	11.4
(Ragu) regular	5-oz. serving	14.0
Mushroom:		
(Prego)	4-oz. serving	22.0
(Prince)	4-oz. serving	11.3
(Ragu)	5-oz. serving	13.0
Canned, dietetic pack		
(Featherweight)	⅔ cup	10.0
*SPAGHETTI SAUCE MIX:		
(Durkee) plain	½ cup	10.4
(French's):		
Italian style	⅝ cup	15.0
Thick homemade style	⅞ cup	24.0
(Spatini)	½ cup	8.4
SPAM, luncheon meat (Hormel):		
Regular or smoke flavored	1-oz. serving	1.1
With cheese chunks	1-oz. serving	.7
Deviled	1-oz. serving	0.
SPECIAL K, cereal (Kellogg's)	1 cup	21.0
SPINACH:		
Fresh, whole leaves	½ cup	.7
Boiled	½ cup	2.8
Canned, regular pack (Sunshine) solids & liq.	½ cup	2.9
Canned, dietetic pack (Featherweight) solids & liq.	½ cup	

Food and Description	Measure or Quantity	Carbohydrates (grams)
Frozen:		
(Birds Eye):		
Chopped or leaf	⅓ of pkg.	3.4
Creamed	⅓ of pkg.	4.9
(Green Giant):		
Creamed	⅓ of pkg.	6.4
Cut leaf, in butter sauce	⅓ of pkg.	4.0
(McKenzie)	⅓ of pkg.	3.0
SQUASH, SUMMER:		
Yellow, boiled slices	½ cup	2.7
Zucchini, boiled slices	½ cup	1.9
Canned (Del Monte) zucchini in tomato sauce	½ cup	7.7
Frozen:		
(Birds Eye)	3⅓ oz.	3.9
(McKenzie) Crookneck	⅓ of pkg.	4.0
(Mrs. Paul's) zucchini, parmesan	⅓ of pkg.	7.0
(Southland) zucchini, sliced	⅕ of 16-oz. pkg.	3.3
SQUASH, WINTER:		
Acorn, baked	½ cup	14.3
Hubbard, baked, mashed	½ cup	11.9
Frozen:		
(Birds Eye)	⅓ of pkg.	9.2
(Southland) butternut	4 oz.	16.0
STEAK & GREEN PEPPERS, frozen:		
(Green Giant)	9-oz. entree	33.2
(Swanson)	8½-oz. entree	12.0
STOCK BASE (French's) beef or chicken	1 tsp.	2.0
STRAWBERRY:		
Fresh, capped	½ cup	6.0
Frozen (Birds Eye):		
Halves	⅓ of pkg.	46.4
Whole	¼ of pkg.	21.3
Whole, quick thaw	½ of pkg.	30.2
STRAWBERRY DRINK (Hi-C):		
Canned	6 fl. oz.	22.0
*Mix	6 fl. oz.	17.0
STRAWBERRY PRESERVE or JAM:		
Sweetened:		
(Smucker's)	1 T.	13.5
(Welch's)	1 T.	13.5
Dietetic or low calorie (See STRAWBERRY SPREAD)		

127

Food and Description	Measure or Quantity	Carbohydrates (grams)
STRAWBERRY SHORTCAKE,		
cereal (General Mills)	1 cup	25.0
STRAWBERRY SPREAD, dietetic:		
(Diet Delight)	1 T.	3.0
(Estee)	1 T.	1.6
(Featherweight) artifically sweetened	1 T.	1.0
(S&W) *Nutradiet*	1 T.	3.0
(Welch's) lite	1 T.	6.2
STUFFING MIX:		
*Chicken, *Stove Top*	½ cup	20.2
*Cornbread, *Stove Top*	½ cup	21.6
Cube (Pepperidge Farm)	1 oz.	22.0
*Pork, *Stove Top*	½ cup	20.3
Seasoned (Pepperidge Farm)	1 oz.	19.9
White bread, *Mrs. Cubbison's*	1 oz.	20.5
STURGEON, smoked	4-oz. serving	0.
SUCCOTASH:		
Canned:		
(Libby's) cream style	½ cup	22.8
(Stokely-Van Camp)	½ cup	17.5
Frozen (Birds Eye)	⅓ of pkg.	20.7
SUGAR:		
Brown	1 T.	12.5
Confectioners'	1 T.	7.7
Granulated	1 T.	11.9
Maple	1¾″ × 1¼″ × ½″ piece	27.0
SUGAR CORN POPS, cereal		
(Kellogg's)	1 cup	26.0
SUGAR CRISP, cereal	⅞ cup	25.6
SUGAR PUFFS, cereal (Malt-O-Meal)	⅞ cup	26.0
SUGAR SMACKS, cereal (Kellogg's)	¾ cup	25.0
SUGAR SUBSTITUTE:		
(Featherweight)	3 drops	0.
Sprinkle Sweet (Pillsbury)	1 tsp.	.5
SUNFLOWER SEED (Fisher):		
In hull, roasted, salted	1 oz.	3.0
Hulled, dry roasted, salted	1 oz.	5.6
Hulled, oil roasted, salted	1 oz.	5.6
SUZY Q (Hostess):		
Banana	1 cake	38.4
Chocolate	1 cake	36.4
SWEETBREADS, calf, braised	4-oz. serving	0.
SWEET POTATO:		
Baked, peeled	5″ × 1″ potato	35.8
Canned, heavy syrup	4-oz. serving	31.2

Food and Description	Measure or Quantity	Carbohydrates (grams)
Frozen (Mrs. Paul's) candied, with apple	4-oz. serving	36.1
*SWEET & SOUR ORIENTAL, canned (La Choy):		
Chicken	7½-oz. serving	50.0
Pork	7½-oz. serving	48.0
SWISS STEAK, frozen (Swanson) *TV Brand*	10-oz. dinner	36.0
SWORDFISH, broiled	3″ × 3″ × ½″ steak	0.
SYRUP (See also TOPPING):		
Regular:		
Apricot (Smucker's)	1 T.	13.0
Blackberry (Smucker's)	1 T.	13.0
Chocolate or chocolate-flavored		
Bosco	1 T.	13.3
(Hershey's)	1 T.	11.7
Corn, *Karo*, dark or light	1 T.	14.6
Maple, *Karo*, imitation	1 T.	14.2
Pancake or waffle:		
(Aunt Jemima)	1 T.	13.1
Golden Griddle	1 T.	13.3
Karo	1 T.	14.4
Log Cabin, regular	1 T.	14.0
Mrs. Butterworth's	1 T.	13.0
Strawberry (Smucker's)	1 T.	13.0
Dietetic or low calorie:		
Blueberry (Featherweight)	1 T.	3.0
Chocolate-flavored (Diet Delight)	1 T.	2.0
Coffee (No-Cal)	1 T.	.4
Cola (No-Cal)	1 T.	Tr.
Maple (S&W) *Nutradiet*	1 T.	3.0
Pancake or waffle:		
(Aunt Jemima)	1 T.	7.3
(Diet Delight)	1 T.	4.0
(Featherweight)	1 T.	3.0
(Tillie Lewis) *Tasti-Diet*	1 T.	1.0

T

TACO:		
*(Ortega)	1 taco	15.0
*Mix (Durkee)	½ cup	3.7
Shell (Ortega)	1 shell	7.7

Food and Description	Measure or Quantity	Carbohydrates (grams)
TAMALE:		
Canned:		
(Hormel) beef, *Short Orders*	7½-oz. can	17.0
(Nalley's) beef	8-oz. serving	25.0
Old El Paso, with chili gravy	1 tamale	11.5
Frozen (Hormel) beef	1 tamale	11.3
TAMALE PIE (Nalley's)	4-oz. serving	12.5
*TANG:		
Grape	6 fl. oz.	23.2
Orange	6 fl. oz.	22.6
TANGERINE or MANDARIN ORANGE:		
Fresh (Sunkist)	1 large tangerine	10.0
Canned, regular pack (Del Monte) solids & liq.	5½-oz. serving	25.3
Canned, dietetic:		
(Diet Delight) Juice pack	½ cup	13.0
(Featherweight) water pack	½ cup	8.0
(S&W) *Nutradiet*	½ cup	7.0
TANGERINE DRINK, canned (Hi-C)	6 fl. oz.	23.0
*TANGERINE JUICE, frozen (Minute Maid)	6 fl. oz.	20.8
TAPIOCA, dry, *Minute,* quick cooking	1 T.	7.9
TAQUITO, frozen (Van de Kamp's) beef	8 oz.	47.0
TARRAGON (French's)	1 tsp.	.7
TASTEEOS, cereal (Ralston Purina)	1¼ cups	22.0
TEA:		
(Lipton):		
Plain	1 teabag	0.
Flavored	1 teabag	<1.0
(Tender Leaf)	1 rounded tsp.	Tr.
TEAM, cereal	1 cup	24.0
TEA MIX, iced:		
*(Lipton) lemon & sugar flavored	1 cup	16.0
**Nestea,* lemon-flavored	8 fl. oz.	.2
TEQUILA SUNRISE COCKTAIL (Mr. Boston) 12½% alcohol	3 fl. oz.	14.4
*TEXTURED VEGETABLE PROTEIN, *Morningstar Farms:*		
Breakfast link	1 link	.3
Breakfast patties	1 patty	3.2
Breakfast strips	1 strip	.2
Grillers	1 pattie	4.5

Food and Description	Measure or Quantity	Carbohydrates (grams)
THURINGER:		
(Hormel):		
Buffet	1-oz. serving	.3
Old Smokehouse	1-oz. serving	.1
(Louis Rich) turkey	1-oz. serving	<1.0
(Oscar Mayer) beef	.8-oz. slice	.7
TIGER TAILS (Hostess)	1 piece	38.9
TOASTER CAKE OR PASTRY:		
Pop-Tarts (Kellogg's):		
Regular:		
Blueberry, brown sugar		
cinnamon & cherry	1 pastry	36.0
Chocolate chip	1 pastry	34.0
Strawberry	1 pastry	37.0
Frosted:		
Blueberry	1 pastry	38.0
Brown sugar cinnamon	1 pastry	34.0
Chocolate-vanilla creme	1 pastry	37.0
Toastettes (Nabisco)	1 pastry	35.0
Toast-R-Cake (Thomas'):		
Blueberry	1 piece	17.7
Bran	1 piece	18.5
Corn	1 piece	17.4
TOASTIES, cereal (Post)	1¼ cup	24.4
TOASTY O's, cereal (Malt-O-Meal)	1¼ cups	20.0
TOMATO:		
Cherry, whole	4 pieces	3.2
Regular, whole	1 med. tomato	7.0
Canned, regular pack:		
(Contadina) sliced	4-oz. serving	10.0
(Del Monte) whole, peeled	8 oz.	10.1
(Stokely-Van Camp) stewed	½ cup	7.5
Canned, dietetic pack:		
(Diet Delight)	½ cup	5.0
(Featherweight)	½ cup	4.0
(S&W) *Nutradiet*, whole	½ cup	5.0
TOMATO JUICE:		
Canned, regular pack:		
(Campbell)	6-fl. oz. can	8.0
(Del Monte)	6-fl.-oz. can	7.4
Musselman's	6 fl. oz.	7.0
Canned, dietetic pack:		
(Diet Delight)	6 fl. oz.	7.0
(Featherweight)	6 fl. oz.	8.0
(S&W) *Nutradiet*	6 fl. oz.	8.0

Food and Description	Measure or Quantity	Carbohydrates (grams)
TOMATO JUICE COCKTAIL:		
(Ocean Spray) *Firehouse Jubilee*	6 fl. oz.	9.1
Snap-E-Tom	6 fl. oz.	7.0
TOMATO PASTE:		
Regular pack:		
(Contadina)	6 oz.	36.0
(Del Monte)	6-oz. can	33.7
(Hunt's)	6-oz. can	30.0
Dietetic (Featherweight) low sodium	6-oz. can	35.0
TOMATO & PEPPER, HOT CHILI		
(Ortega) Jalapeno	1-oz. serving	1.1
TOMATO, PICKLED (Claussen)		
green	1 piece	1.1
TOMATO PUREE, canned:		
Regular (Contadina) heavy	1 cup	22.0
Dietetic (Featherweight)	1 cup	20.0
TOMATO SAUCE, canned:		
(Contadina) regular	1 cup	18.0
(Del Monte):		
Regular	1 cup	17.0
Hot	1 cup	17.0
With tomato tidbits	1 cup	19.0
(Hunt's) with cheese	4-oz. serving	10.0
TOM COLLINS, canned (Mr. Boston) 12½% alcohol	3 fl. oz.	10.8
TONGUE, beef, braised	4-oz. serving	.5
TOPPING:		
Regular:		
Butterscotch (Smucker's)	1 T.	16.5
Caramel (Smucker's)	1 T.	16.5
Chocolate fudge (Hershey's)	1 T.	7.3
Pecans in syrup (Smucker's)	1 T.	14.0
Pineapple (Smucker's)	1 T.	16.0
Dietetic, chocolate (Tillie Lewis) *Tasti-Diet*	1 T.	2.0
TOPPING, WHIPPED:		
Regular:		
Cool Whip (Birds Eye), dairy	1 T.	1.2
Lucky Whip, aerosol	1 T.	.5
Whip Topping (Rich's)	¼ oz.	1.2
Dietetic (Featherweight)	1 T.	.5
*Mix:		
Regular, *Dream Whip*	1 T.	1.0
Dietetic (D-Zerta)	1 T.	.3
TOP RAMEN, beef (Nissin Foods)	3-oz. serving	50.5
TORTILLA (Amigos)	6″ × ⅛″ tortilla	19.7

Food and Description	Measure or Quantity	Carbohydrates (grams)
TOSTADA, frozen (Van de Kamp's)	8½ oz.	37.0
TOSTADA SHELL (Ortega)	1 shell	6.0
TOTAL, cereal, regular	1 cup	23.0
TRIPE, canned (Libby's)	6-oz. serving	1.1
TRIX, cereal (General Mills)	1 cup	25.0
TUNA	any quantity	0.
TUNA HELPER (General Mills:		
Country dumplings or creamy		
noodles	⅕ of pkg.	31.0
Noodles & cheese sauce	⅕ of pkg.	28.0
TUNA NOODLE CASSEROLE,		
frozen (Stouffer's)	5¾-oz. serving	18.0
TUNA PIE, frozen:		
(Banquet)	8-oz. pie	42.7
(Morton)	8-oz. pie	36.4
TUNA SALAD:		
Home recipe	4-oz. serving	4.0
Canned (Carnation)	¼ of 7½ oz. can	3.3
TURKEY:		
Raw	any quantity	0.
Canned:		
(Hormel) chunk	6¾-oz. serving	.6
Packaged:		
(Eckrich) sliced	1-oz. serving	1.3
(Hormel) breast	.8-oz. slice	.1
(Louis Rich):		
Turkey bologna	1-oz. slice	1.0
Turkey cotto salami	1-oz. slice	<1.0
Turkey ham, chopped	1-oz. slice	<1.0
Turkey pastrami	1-oz. slice	<1.0
(Oscar Mayer) breast	¾-oz. slice	0.
Roasted	any quantity	0.
Smoked (Louis Rich):		
Drumsticks	1 oz. (without bone)	<1.0
Wing drumettes	1 oz. (without bone)	<1.0
TURKEY DINNER OR ENTREE,		
frozen:		
(Banquet):		
Regular	11-oz. dinner	27.8
Man Pleaser	19-oz. dinner	73.8
(Green Giant)	9-oz. entree	36.6
(Swanson):		
Regular with gravy & dressing	9¼-oz. entree	25.0
Hungry Man	18¾-oz. dinner	70.0

Food and Description	Measure or Quantity	Carbohydrates (grams)
TV Brand (Weight Watchers) sliced, 3-compartment	11½-oz. dinner	40.0
	15¼-oz. meal	37.3
TURKEY PIE, frozen:		
(Banquet):		
Regular	8-oz. pie	40.6
Supreme	8-oz. pie	41.0
(Stouffer's)	10-oz. pie	35.0
(Swanson):		
Regular	8-oz. pie	39.0
Hungry Man	1-lb. pie	61.0
TURKEY TETRAZINI, frozen:		
(Stouffer's)	6-oz. serving	16.9
(Weight Watchers)	13-oz. bag	36.9
TURMERIC (French's)	1 tsp.	1.3
TURNIP GREENS, canned		
(Sunshine) chopped, solids & liq.	½ cup	2.5
TURNOVER:		
Frozen (Pepperidge Farm):		
Apple	1 turnover	35.0
Blueberry or cherry	1 turnover	32.0
Peach	1 turnover	34.0
Raspberry	1 turnover	37.0
Refrigerated (Pillsbury):		
Apple	1 turnover	23.0
Cherry	1 turnover	24.0
TWINKIE (Hostess):		
Regular	1 cake	26.0
Devil's food	1 cake	24.7

V

VALPOLICELLA WINE (Antinori)	3 fl. oz.	6.3
VANDERMINT, liqueur	1 fl. oz.	10.2
VEAL	any quantity	0.
VEAL DINNER, frozen:		
(Banquet) parmigiana	11-oz. dinner	42.1
(Swanson)		
Hungry Man, parmigiana	20½-oz. dinner	70.0
TV Brand, parmigiana	12¼-oz. dinner	41.0
(Weight Watchers) parmigiana, 2-compartment	9-oz. meal	12.0
VEAL STEAK, frozen (Hormel):		
Regular	4-oz. serving	2.1

134

Food and Description	Measure or Quantity	Carbohydrates (grams)
Breaded	4-oz. serving	13.1
VEGETABLE JUICE COCKTAIL:		
Regular, *V-8*	6 fl. oz.	8.0
Dietetic:		
(S&W) *Nutradiet*, low sodium	6 fl. oz.	8.0
V-8, low sodium	6 fl. oz.	9.0
VEGETABLES, MIXED:		
Canned, regular pack:		
(Del Monte) drained	½ cup	9.2
(La Choy):		
Chinese	1 cup	1.6
Chop Suey	1 cup	6.9
Canned, dietetic pack		
(Featherweight)	½ cup	8.0
Frozen:		
(Birds Eye):		
Regular:		
Broccoli, cauliflower & carrots in cheese sauce	3⅓ oz.	7.5
Mixed	3⅓ oz.	13.3
Pea & cauliflower with cream sauce	3⅓ oz.	13.6
Pea & pearl onion	3⅓ oz.	13.5
Stew	6.7	22.1
Blue Ribbon:		
Broccoli, carrots & pasta in lightly seasoned sauce	3⅓ oz.	10.5
Corn, green beans & pasta in lightly seasoned sauce	3⅓ oz.	14.9
Mixed	3⅓ oz.	19.3
Farm Fresh:		
Broccoli, cauliflower & carrot strips	3.2 oz.	5.1
Broccoli, corn & red pepper	3.2 oz.	10.9
Brussels sprouts, cauliflower & carrots	3.2 oz.	6.1
International Style:		
Chinese style	⅓ of pkg.	8.4
Italian style	⅓ of pkg.	13.9
Japanese style	⅓ of pkg.	10.4
Mexican style	⅓ of pkg.	16.1
Stir Fry:		
Cantonese style	⅓ of pkg.	11.4
Chinese style	⅓ of pkg.	6.9
Japanese style	⅓ of pkg.	5.9

Food and Description	Measure or Quantity	Carbohydrates (grams)
(Green Giant):		
Regular:		
Broccoli, cauliflower, carrots in cheese sauce	3⅓ oz.	7.1
Mixed	3⅓ oz.	12.3
Pea, pea pod & water chestnuts in butter sauce	3 oz.	7.5
Harvest Fresh	4-oz.	13.3
Harvest Get Togethers:		
Broccoli-cauliflower medley	3⅓-oz.	8.3
Cauliflower-carrot bonanza	3⅓-oz.	6.0
Japanese style	3⅓-oz.	5.8
(La Choy):		
Chinese	5-oz. serving	5.3
Japanese	5-oz. serving	5.8
(McKenzie)	3⅓-oz.	13.0
(Southland):		
California blend	⅕ of. 16-oz. pkg	7.0
VEGETABLES IN PASTRY, frozen		
(Pepperidge Farm):		
Asparagus with mornay sauce	3¾-oz.	18.0
Broccoli with cheese, mushrooms dijon or spinach almondine	3¾-oz.	19.0
Zucchini provencal	3¾-oz.	21.0
VEGETABLE STEW, canned, *Dinty Moore*	7½-oz. serving	18.3
"VEGETARIAN FOODS":		
Canned or dry:		
Chicken, fried (Loma Linda) with gravy	1½-oz. piece	1.9
Chili (Worthington)	¼ can (5-oz. serving)	20.0
Choplet (Worthington)	1 choplet	3.0
Dinner cuts (Loma Linda) drained	1 cut	1.6
Franks, big (Loma Linda)	1.9-oz. frank	4.1
Franks, sizzle (Loma Linda)	2.2-oz. frank	4.6
FriChik (Worthington)	1 piece	1.0
Granburger (Worthington)	6 T.	12.0
Little links (Loma Linda) drained	.8-oz. link	1.3
Non-meatballs (Worthington)	1 meatball	7.6
Nuteena (Loma Linda)	½" slice	7.6
Proteena (Loma Linda)	½" slice	6.5
Sandwich spread:		
(Loma Linda)	1 T.	1.7
(Worthington)	2½-oz.	2.0

Food and Description	Measure or Quantity	Carbohydrates (grams)
Savorex (Loma Linda)	1 T.	2.0
Soyalac (Loma Linda):		
I-soyalac	1 cup	17.0
Concentrate, liquid	1 cup	33.8
Ready to use	1 cup	15.9
Soyameat (Worthington):		
Sliced beef	1 slice	1.5
Diced chicken	¼ cup	2.0
Sliced chicken	1 slice	1.0
Salisbury steak	1 slice	2.0
Soyamel, any kind (Worthington)	1 oz.	15.2
Stew pack (Loma Linda) drained	1 piece	.6
Super links (Worthington)	1 link	4.0
Swiss steak with gravy (Loma Linda)	1 steak	8.9
Tender bits (Loma Linda) drained	1 piece	1.1
Vege-burger (Loma Linda) no salt added	½ cup	6.9
Vegelona (Loma Linda)	½" slice	7.0
Vega-links (Worthington)	1 link	1.5
Wheat protein	4 oz.	10.0
Worthington 209	1 slice	1.5
Frozen:		
Beef-like slices (Worthington)	1 slice	2.0
Beef pie (Worthington)	1 pie	51.0
Bologna (Loma Linda)	1 oz.	2.8
Chicken (Loma Linda)	1 slice	1.5
Chicken, fried (Loma Linda)	2-oz. serving	3.6
Chicken pie (Worthington)	1 pie	42.0
Chic-Ketts (Worthington)	½ cup	6.0
Corned beef, loaf, or sliced (Worthington)	2½-oz.	6.0
FriPats (Worthington)	1 pat	3.0
Meatballs (Loma Linda)	1 meatball	2.2
Prosage (Worthington)	1 link	1.7
Roast Beef (Loma Linda)	1-oz.	1.3
Sausage, breakfast (Loma Linda)	⅓" slice	1.4
Smoked beef, roll (Worthington)	2½-oz.	7.0
Turkey (Loma Linda)	1-oz.	1.6
Wham, roll (Worthington)	2½-oz.	4.0
VERMOUTH:		
Dry & extra dry (Lejon; Noilly Pratt)	1 fl. oz.	.7
Sweet (Lejon; Taylor)	1 fl. oz.	3.8
VICHY WATER (Schweppes)	any quantity	0.

Food and Description	Measure or Quantity	Carbohydrates (grams)
VIENNA SAUSAGE:		
(Hormel):		
Regular	1 sausage	Tr.
Chicken	1-oz. serving	.2
(Libby's):		
In barbecue sauce	2½-oz.	2.0
In beef broth	1 link	.3
VINEGAR	1 T.	.9

W

Food and Description	Measure or Quantity	Carbohydrates (grams)
WAFFLE, frozen:		
(Aunt Jemima) jumbo	1 waffle	14.5
(Eggo):		
Blueberry or strawberry	1 waffle	18.0
Home style	1 waffle	17.0
(Roman Meal)	1 waffle	16.5
WALLBANGER COCKTAIL, canned		
(Mr. Boston) 12½% alcohol	3 fl. oz	
WALNUT, English or Persian		
(Diamond A)	1 cup	12.8
WATER CHESTNUT, canned:		
(Chun King) solids & liq.	8½-oz. can	22.0
(La Choy) drained	¼ of 8-oz. can	3.9
WATERCRESS, trimmed	½ cup	.5
WATERMELON:		
Wedge	4″ × 8″ wedge	27.3
Diced	½ cup	5.1
WELSH RAREBIT:		
Home recipe	1 cup	14.6
Frozen:		
(Green Giant)	5-oz. serving	11.4
(Stouffer's)	5-oz. serving	17.0
WESTERN DINNER, frozen:		
(Banquet)	11-oz. dinner	32.4
(Morton) *Round-Up*	11.8-oz. dinner	33.5
(Swanson):		
Hungry Man	17¾-oz. dinner	73.0
TV Brand	11¾-oz. dinner	45.0
WHEATENA, cereal	¼-cup	22.5
WHEAT FLAKES CEREAL:		
(Breakfast Best)	1 cup	30.3
(Featherweight)	1¼ cup	23.0
(Van Brode)	¾ cup	22.7

Food and Description	Measure or Quantity	Carbohydrates (grams)
WHEAT GERM, RAW (Elam's)	1-oz.	12.8
WHEAT GERM CEREAL (Kretschmer):		
Regular	¼ cup	8.8
Brown sugar & honey	¼ cup	17.0
WHEAT HEARTS, cereal (General Mills)	1 oz.	21.0
WHEATIES, cereal	1 cup	23.0
WHEAT & OATMEAL, cereal, hot (Elam's)	1 oz.	18.8
WHITE CASTLE:		
Bun only	.8-oz	12.4
Cheeseburger (meat & cheese only)	1.54-oz. serving	5.2
Fish sandwich (fish only without tartar sauce)	1.48-oz. serving	7.8
French fries	2.6-oz. serving	15.1
Hamburger (meat only, no bun)	1.2-oz. serving	5.2
WHITE FISH, LAKE:		
Baked, stuffed	4-oz.	6.6
Smoked	4-oz.	0.
WILD BERRY DRINK, canned (Hi-C)	6 fl. oz.	22.0
WINCHELL'S DONUT HOUSE:		
Buttermilk, old fashioned	2-oz. piece	56.0
Cake, devil's food, iced	2-oz. piece	54.0
Cake, white, donut-hole	.4-oz. piece	45.2
Raised, apple-fritter	4¼-oz. piece	48.8
Raised, glazed	1¾-oz. piece	48.5
WINE, COOKING (Regina):		
Burgundy or sauterne	¼ cup	Tr.
Sherry	¼ cup	5.0

Y

Food and Description	Measure or Quantity	Carbohydrates (grams)
YEAST, BAKER'S (Fleischmann's):		
Dry, active	¼-oz.	2.7
Fresh & household, active	.6-oz. cake	2.0
YOGURT:		
Regular:		
Plain:		
(Bison)	.8-oz. container	16.8
(Colombo):		
Regular	8-oz. container	13.0
Natural Lite	8-oz. container	17.0

Food and Description	Measure or Quantity	Carbohydrates (grams)
(Dannon)	8-oz. container	17.0
(Friendship)	8-oz. container	15.0
Yoplait	6-oz. container	14.0
Plain with honey, *Yoplait, Custard Style*	6-oz. container	23.0
Apple:		
(Colombo) spiced	8-oz. container	39.0
(Dannon) Dutch	8-oz. container	49.0
Mélangé	6-oz. container	31.0
Yoplait (General Mills)	6-oz. container	32.0
Apricot:		
(Bison)	8-oz. container	45.9
Banana (Dannon)	8-oz. container	49.0
Banana-strawberry (Colombo)	8-oz container	38.0
Berry, *Yoplait, Breakfast Yogurt*	6-oz. container	39.0
Blueberry:		
(Bison):		
Regular	8-oz. container	45.9
Light	6-oz. container	28.1
(Colombo)	8-oz. container	38.0
(Dannon)	8-oz. container	49.0
(Friendship)	8-oz. container	57.0
Mélangé	6-oz. container	31.0
(New Country) ripple	8-oz. container	43.0
(Sweet'n Low)	8-oz. container	33.0
Yoplait (General Mills)	6-oz. container	32.0
Boysenberry		
(Bison)	8-oz. container	45.9
(Dannon)	8-oz. container	49.0
(Sweet'n Low)	8-oz. container	33.0
Cherry:		
(Bison) Light	6-oz. container	28.1
(Colombo) black	8-oz. container	34.0
(Dannon)	8-oz. container	49.0
(Friendship)	8-oz. container	57.0
Mélangé	6-oz. container	31.0
(Sweet'n Low)	8-oz. container	33.0
Yoplait	6-oz. container	32.0
Cherry-vanilla (Colombo)	8-oz. container	40.0
Citrus, *Yoplait, Breakfast Yogurt*	6-oz. container	43.0
Coffee (Colombo; Dannon)	8-oz. container	29.0
Date-Walnut-Raisin (Bison)	8-oz. container	45.9
Fruit Crunch (New Country)	8-oz. container	40.0
Granola Strawberry (Colombo)	8-oz. container	40.0
Guava (Dannon)	8-oz. container	40.0
Hawaiian salad (New Country)	8-oz. container	40.0

Food and Description	Measure or Quantity	Carbohydrates (grams)
Honey vanilla (Colombo)	8-oz. container	30.0
Lemon:		
(Dannon)	8-oz. container	32.0
(Sweet'N Low)	8-oz. container	33.0
Yoplait:		
Regular	6-oz. container	32.0
Custard style	6-oz. container	30.0
Orange, *Yoplait*	6-oz. container	32.0
Orchard, *Yoplait, Breakfast*		
Yogurt	6-oz. container	40.0
Peach:		
(Bison)	8-oz. container	45.9
(Dannon)	8-oz. container	49.0
(Friendship)	8-oz. container	57.0
(New Country) 'N Cream	8-oz. container	40.0
(Sweet'N Low)	8-oz. container	33.0
Peach Melba (Colombo)	8-oz. container	37.0
Piña Colada:		
(Colombo)	8-oz. container	40.0
(Dannon)	8-oz. container	49.0
(Friendship)	8-oz. container	57.0
Pineapple:		
(Bison) Light	6-oz. container	28.1
Mélangé	6-oz. container	31.0
Raspberry:		
(Dannon) red	8-oz. container	49.0
(Friendship)	8-oz. container	57.0
Mélangé	6-oz. container	31.0
(Sweet'N Low)	8-oz. container	33.0
Yoplait	6-oz. container	32.0
Yoplait, Custard Style	6-oz. container	30.0
Strawberry:		
(Bison) light	6-oz. container	28.1
(Colombo)	8-oz. container	36.0
(Dannon)	8-oz. container	49.0
(Friendship)	8-oz. container	57.0
Mélangé	6-oz. container	31.0
(Sweet'N Low)	8-oz. container	33.0
Yoplait	6-oz. container	32.0
Strawberry banana (Sweet'N Low)	8-oz. container	33.0
Strawberry colada (Colombo)	8-oz. container	36.0
Tropical fruit (Sweet'N Low)	8-oz. container	33.0
Vanilla:		
(Dannon)	8-oz. container	32.0
(New Country) French, ripple	8-oz. container	40.0

Food and Description	Measure or Quantity	Carbohydrates (grams)
Frozen, hard:		
Banana:		
Danny-Yo	3½-oz. serving	21.0
Danny-in-a-Cup	8-oz. cup	42.0
Boysenberry:		
Danny-on-a-Stick, carob coated	2½-fl.-oz. bar	13.0
Danny-Yo	3½-oz. serving	21.0
Boysenberry swirl (Bison)	¼ of 16-oz. container	24.0
Cherry vanilla (Bison)	¼ of 16-oz. container	24.0
Chocolate:		
(Bison)	¼ of 16-oz. container	24.0
(Colombo) bar, chocolate coated	1 bar	17.0
(Dannon):		
Danny-in-a-Cup	8-fl.-oz. cup	42.0
Danny-on-a-Stick, chocolate coated	2½-fl.-oz. bar	13.0
Chocolate chip (Bison)	¼ of 16-oz. container	24.0
Chocolate chocolate chip (Colombo)	4-oz. serving	28.0
Mocha (Colombo) bar	1 bar	14.0
Piña Colada:		
(Colombo)	4-oz. serving	20.0
(Dannon):		
Danny-in-a-Cup	8-oz. cup	42.0
Danny-on-a-Stick	2½-fl.-oz. bar	13.0
Raspberry, red (Dannon)		
Danny-on-a-Stick, chocolate coated	2½-fl. oz. bar	13.0
Danny-in-a-Cup	8-oz. container	42.0
Danny-Yo	3½ fl. oz.	21.0
Raspberry swirl (Bison)	¼ of 16-oz. container	24.0
Strawberry:		
(Bison)	¼ of 16-oz. container	24.0
(Colombo):		
Regular	4-oz. serving	20.0
Bar	1 bar	14.0
(Dannon):		
Danny-in-a-Cup	8 fl. oz.	42.0
Danny-Yo	3½ fl. oz.	21.0
Vanilla:		
(Bison)	¼ of 16-oz. container	24.0
(Colombo):		
Regular	4-oz. serving	20.0

Food and Description	Measure or Quantity	Carbohydrates (grams)
Bar, chocolate covered (Dannon):	1 bar	17.0
Danny-in-a-Cup	8 fl. oz.	20.0
Danny-on-a-Stick	2½-fl.-oz. bar	13.0
Danny-Yo	3½-oz. serving	21.0
Frozen, soft (Colombo)	6-fl.-oz. serving	24.0

Z

ZINFANDEL WINE (Inglenook)		
Vintage	3 fl. oz.	.3
ZITI, frozen (Weight Watchers)	12½-oz. pkg.	41.2
ZWIEBACK (Gerber; Nabisco)	1 piece	5.0

SIGNET Books of Special Interest

Staying Healthy with SIGNET Books